WITCHES,

WESTERNERS,

and HIV

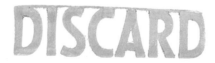

WITCHES, WESTERNERS, and HIV

Alexander Rödlach

AIDS & Cultures of Blame in Africa

Left Coast Press Inc.

Walnut Creek, CA

LEFT COAST PRESS, INC.
1630 North Main Street, #400
Walnut Creek, CA 94596
http://www.LCoastPress.com

Library of Congress Cataloging-in-Publication Data
Rödlach, Alexander.
  Witches, Westerners, and HIV : AIDS and cultures of blame in Africa / Alexander Rödlach.
      p.   cm.
  Includes bibliographical references and index.
  ISBN 1-59874-033-4 (hardback: alk. paper)—ISBN 1-59874-034-2 (pbk.: alk. paper)
  1. Medical anthropology—Zimbabwe.   2. AIDS (Disease)—Zimbabwe—Public opinion.
  3. HIV infections—Zimbabwe—Public opinion.   4. Conspiracies—Zimbabwe.   5. Witchcraft—
  Zimbabwe.   6. Public opinion—Zimbabwe.   7. Zimbabwe—Social life and customs   I. Title.
  GN296.5.Z55R63 2006
  306.4'61096891—dc22   2006019726

Printed in the United States of America

This paper is acid free and meets the minimum requirements of ANSI/NISCO Z39.48-1992 (R 1997) (Permanence of Paper).

Cover: The two figures on the cover were carved by the Zimbabwean artist, Mr. Sheunesu Shumba. The left figure shows a man staring ahead squatting on the ground, the head supported by arms resting on the knees. He represents a Zimbabwean pondering the dire conditions his country is facing, including the AIDS epidemic, that make his and his contemporaries' life so miserable. He asks himself why he has to suffer so much. The figure on the right side shows a man sitting on a drum trying to find answers to the same startling question. He represents a traditional diviner calling the ancestors expecting them to provide him with answers. The photos of the carvings were taken by Heinz Helf.

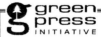

KM Empires is committed to preserving ancient forests and natural resources. We elected to print *Empire on the Horizon* on 50% post consumer recycled paper, processed chlorine free. As a result, for this printing, we have saved:

306 trees (40' tall and 6-8" diameter)
130,446 gallons of water
52,461 kilowatt hours of electricity
14,382 pounds of solid waste
28,251 pounds of greenhouse gases

KM Empires made this paper choice because our printer, Thomson-Shore, Inc., is a member of Green Press Initiative, a nonprofit program dedicated to supporting authors, publishers, and suppliers in their efforts to reduce their use of fiber obtained from endangered forests.

For more information, visit www.greenpressinitiative.org

Text design by Detta Penna

06 07 08 09 10 5 4 3 2 1

Contents

Acknowledgments

There is a saying among the Zimbabwean Ndebele that "the ungrateful is a witch" (*ongabongiyo ngumthakathi*). I am indebted to the many persons who contributed to writing this book.

I owe special thanks to Gerald Murray and Russ Bernard for their scholarly advice before, during, and after the preparation of my doctoral dissertation in cultural anthropology, which served as the starting point for this book. I thank the Center of African Studies and the Department of Anthropology at the University of Florida for various grants and assistantships, and the National Science Foundation and the Society of the Divine Word for funding my field research.

I deeply appreciate the kindness and warmth of many Zimbabweans. I gratefully acknowledge the help of Michael Bourdillon of the department of sociology at the University of Zimbabwe in Harare, and of Riitta Dlodlo, then the director of health services of Bulawayo, for facilitating the necessary Zimbabwean paperwork for conducting field research. My gratitude goes to Roland Altmannsberger, Bruce Ehlers, Thadeusz Grenda, Zbigniew Oldynski, Alphons Schoepf, Ben Strydom, Krystian Traczyk, and the Presentation Sisters in Harare for solving logistical problems during my field research in Zimbabwe. During the fieldwork, my landlady Ursula Murray actively supported the study by searching the Bulawayo libraries and archives. She did this together with another volunteer, Val Deas, a retired school teacher. Josina Mpofu, who helped with the household, was an excellent source of information; often I began to comprehend certain issues after a chat with her. Especially in the early days, the home-based caregivers in the township took me with them on house calls, which enabled me to observe the impact of HIV/AIDS on the patient and the family. Members of the Catholic parishes in Nkulumane and Plumtree welcomed me "with both hands"—*ngezandla zombili*, as the Ndebele say. Special thanks go to Mrs. Chuma, Monica Manenge, Fabian Sibelo, and Mrs. Tshuma.

Crucial to the success of the study was working together with assistants, particularly Bernadette Maphosa, Eddie Dzinda Ngoma, and Reuben Alven Ngwenya. Saliwe Phiri, Sola Dube, Rachel Mukau, Elizabeth Mutizwa, Onesimo Matsvaire, and Sithandokuhle Ndlovu spent many hours administering the survey. During the first months of the study, a group of baccalaureate students from the National University of Science and Technology were involved in collecting data through methods from cognitive anthropology: Mr. Banga, Mavis Chikwena, Tichaona Gapu, Chiedza Makamure, A. Matayi, Albert Murwira, Thomas Mutswiti, Farai Mutyasera, Cheneso Muvandi, Tsitsi Ndoro, H. V. Nyapokoto, Simbiso Rukatya, Ronald Alfred Sithole, Chipo Takawira, Thembiso Tembani. Jabulani Mthombeni and Kiaratiwa Sibelo spent much of their time meticulously transcribing the taped interviews. Carmen Luphahla and Beauty Nyathi were helpful in selecting knowledgeable informants.

I am indebted to my colleagues at the Anthropos Institute, who provided me with time and space to write this book, and to Jeanne Weismantel, who did its first thorough editing. I also wish to thank Left Coast Press for recognizing the significance of the original book proposal. Jennifer Collier, their senior editor, has been a pleasant, thoughtful, and efficient person with whom to work. My gratitude goes to Judy Johnstone, who painstakingly edited the text, and to Detta Penna, who managed the production process and designed the book.

To all those who were mentioned and to the many others, I express my sincere gratitude for their inspiration, motivation, and support.

Thank you!

Siyabonga!

Taboka!

Tinotenda!

Introduction

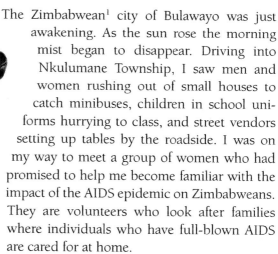

The Zimbabwean[1] city of Bulawayo was just awakening. As the sun rose the morning mist began to disappear. Driving into Nkulumane Township, I saw men and women rushing out of small houses to catch minibuses, children in school uniforms hurrying to class, and street vendors setting up tables by the roadside. I was on my way to meet a group of women who had promised to help me become familiar with the impact of the AIDS epidemic on Zimbabweans. They are volunteers who look after families where individuals who have full-blown AIDS are cared for at home.

Zimbabwe, like many African countries, is hard hit by the AIDS epidemic. In many houses of Nkulumane Township there was at least one person suffering from the disease. Most families could not afford to have sick members treated in a hospital. Instead, they tried their best to ease the suffering at home. Often spouses and elderly parents carried the burden of care. They washed the patients several times a day—necessary because of the persistent diarrhea that accompanies AIDS. They spoon-fed patients unable to feed themselves and, if they could

1

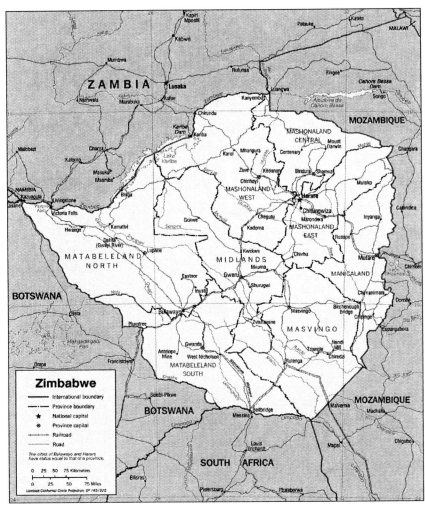

Map of Zimbabwe. (Perry-Castaneda Library Map Collection, University of Texas at Austin)

afford to purchase medications, administered them; however, most of them did not have the necessary funds. Often the only outside support was provided by groups like the one I was joining today, the so-called home-based caregivers.

We met at the local Catholic Church and walked together along dusty roads. As we approached the first house, I spotted a piece of red cloth on the front fence. The red cloth is, in most of southern Africa, an indicator to neighbors and passersby that the family who lives there has lost a member, and an invitation to enter and grieve with them. Nearing, we could see that the curtains and furniture had already been removed from some of the rooms, as prescribed by local custom, to provide space for the people who would congregate to console the bereaved family. The news of the death must have been recent because we did not hear mournful singing of women from the house, nor were visiting men sitting in the yard. My companions realized that their patient had died. They spoke kindly to the family, offering condolences and *inyembezi* (literal meaning, "tears"), a small token meant to help with funeral expenses.

Promising to return later, we then called on a man in his early thirties. His three young children greeted us in the front yard. They were supposed to be in school, but household funds had been drained by the man's illness, and no money was available for school uniforms and fees. Standing in the entrance, I saw only an old sofa and small table in the sitting room; a few yellowed magazine cuttings decorated the rough walls. It appeared that family belongings had been sold to pay for the man's treatment.

The foul odor was common in households with AIDS patients suffering persistent diarrhea. Even frequent washing of soiled clothes and blankets cannot remove the odor. We heard the man coughing in another room. His wife, visibly worn out from months of caring for him, ushered us in to see her husband. We were looking at a man exhausted from physical suffering who had lost all hope of improvement. He appeared depressed as his family faced poverty and starvation. The home-based caregivers consoled him through their prayers and left behind some painkillers, disinfectants, and ointments. They gave the wife a few food items and some laundry soap and promised to try to get the children back in school. Knowing it fell far short of what was needed, the women gave what they could.

Looking at me, the man asked "Why do I have to suffer so much? Why is the suffering of Zimbabweans and other Africans so extreme, compared to people elsewhere? Who is responsible for this?" He was not alone in posing such questions. During my years in Zimbabwe, I frequently heard these questions. The deep suffering and desperation caused by AIDS is painfully and lyrically expressed in several songs by renowned Zimbabwean musician Oliver Mtukudzi. In the song *Todii ne AIDS*? ("What Shall We Do About AIDS?") he struggles, as do so many people in Zimbabwe and elsewhere, to make sense of the suffering and to answer persistently elusive questions: Why has HIV/AIDS caused so much pain? What is the origin of the disease? Will we ever stop its spread? How can we support, and eventually cure, those who are suffering?

Living and working amid the epidemic in Zimbabwe for many years, I became intrigued by people's search for answers and by their interpretations of the disease. People found answers that were credible to them. Many times they suspected various malicious agents, usually hidden from view, to be the instigators of their suffering. They pointed fingers at suspected persons. I began to study the processes underlying the attribution of meanings to HIV/AIDS, particularly two types—sorcery[2] beliefs and conspiracy theories—that featured prominently in my discussions with Zimbabweans. This research became a point of entry for me into the global and comparative questions of how these two types of beliefs become attached to the disease, attributing the epidemic with meaning and shaping behavior.

While each culture, nation, and locality affected by AIDS creates its own nexus of meaning, there are crucial similarities. These shared processes and meanings have important implications for our theoretical understanding of AIDS, as well as for the practical and increasingly critical work of treating and reversing the epidemic.

The search for meaning in the face of misfortune is a fundamental human quest, in evidence across cultures and widely researched by social scientists. Understandings of disease produced by this search for meaning do not necessarily match biomedical explanations. This is reflected in the classic distinction between *disease*, which refers to abnormalities in the structure and function of body organs and symptoms, and *illness*, which refers to the human experience of sickness that is shaped by cultural factors governing perception, labeling, explanation, and valuation of the discomforting experience (Kleinman et al. 1978:251–52; Kleinman 1980:72). While the first is mainly the realm of biomedical discourse, the latter encompasses various popular conceptualizations of sickness.

The distinction between disease and illness has been widely applied to the AIDS epidemic and many studies focusing specifically on the *illness* aspect of HIV/AIDS have been conducted globally since the beginning of the epidemic.[3] Illness studies have described several categories of popular beliefs about HIV-infection and AIDS. Aggleton and colleagues (1989:57) describe (1) beliefs about AIDS itself, what it is and how it can be diagnosed, (2) other beliefs that "explain" the origin of AIDS and why some people develop AIDS while others do not, (3) related beliefs that identify the people, situations, and activities perceived to be particularly risky, and finally (4) those beliefs that create distinctions between supposedly "innocent" and "guilty" victims of infection. I focus on the second category, namely causal explanations of the origin and genesis of the epidemic as well as the reasons particular individuals get sick as opposed to others. In cultures around the world, belief in sorcery and conspiracy theories represents a way in which people make sense of the origin and spread of AIDS. Unfortunately, they are frequently the least understood by social and medical workers, policymakers, and others on whom care and prevention depends.

These two types of belief have a common premise: they attribute *blame* for misfortune in general and disease in particular. This blame reaction is at the core of all sorcery beliefs and conspiracy theories (e.g., Graubard 1984:240); some scholars argue that blame is a natural tendency in human society (e.g., Briggs 1996a:61). Blame attributed to some malicious agent is a personalistic illness explanation (Glick 1967:775; Mitchell 1960:194). In the case of HIV/AIDS, a broad body of research documents cases in which the disease is thought to be the outcome of a deliberate plot by some kind of problematic "other"—another race, class, or ethnic group, or simply a person who is somewhat different.[4]

Of course, these two types of beliefs were not the only meanings attached to the AIDS epidemic; my research unearthed a wide range of highly diverse beliefs explaining why certain individuals and racial or ethnic groups are more likely to become infected than others, why the AIDS epidemic is more widespread in certain countries and geographical regions than in others, and why treatment and cure are unavailable to them or nonexistent in Zimbabwe.

As people actively construct meaning around AIDS, they produce a rich diversity of causal explanations. These range from sexual transmission, lack of hygiene, loss of cultural values, and divine or ancestral punishment, to causes related to political and economic conditions (see Rödlach 2005). However, it became clear to me that even people who expressed very different explanations for the disease simultaneously attributed either sorcery or a conspiracy, or both, to the illness or AIDS-related symptoms of particular individuals and to the fact that no treatment is available.

This book argues that individuals can simultaneously, or at least consecutively, espouse personalistic and non-personalistic explanations. Intrigued by the high incidence of sorcery suspicions and conspiracy theories, combined with the tendency of individuals to alternate between various discourses that I encountered during fieldwork in Zimbabwe, I later refined, expanded, and generalized the Zimbabwean case study in order to make arguments of cross-cultural import.

In 1991 I arrived in Plumtree, a small town with a few thousand residents located on the southwestern border of Zimbabwe. Plumtree developed around a railway station, has several schools and a hospital, and is the administrative center of the area. The town became my community, and its residents my companions, for the following two years. They welcomed me into their households, introduced me to their families and friends, patiently taught me their language, and helped me become acquainted with their beliefs, values, and customs. I was, however, not a regular companion for them; I came to Zimbabwe as a Catholic priest working in the local Catholic Church.

I left Plumtree in 1993 when I was assigned to a church in a township in Bulawayo, the second largest city of Zimbabwe, about one hundred kilometers northeast of Plumtree. There I lived and worked until 1998, when I left Zimbabwe to pursue graduate studies in cultural anthropology. In 2001 and for the whole of 2003 I returned to Plumtree and Bulawayo to conduct ethnographic fieldwork.

Although I became fluent in Ndebele,[5] the commonly used local language in the area, and was even given an Ndebele clan name, I remained a stranger to Zimbabweans. From their perspective, I looked different from them, I behaved oddly at times, and I spoke their language with a funny accent (as the children told me bluntly). Living with them for several years, with their continual assistance, I was able to develop a deep understanding of their aspirations and fears, their joys and difficulties, and the way they view their world. I became aware how strongly southern Zimbabweans relate their well-being and health to their relationship with others and to supernatural forces.

Zimbabweans commonly believe that if these relationships are "healthy" they will be prosperous and enjoy physical and mental health; however, when relationships go sour they result in misfortune and ill health. Continual bad luck, serious health problems, and even death were attributed to occult forces by some who had experienced such suffering. People tried hard to identify problems in their relationships in order to explain their difficulties. If other individuals were found to be responsible, avenues could be pursued to counteract the evil works of such people.

Throughout my years of priestly ministry I had ample opportunities to observe these dynamics. Many Zimbabweans told me confidentially and in prayers, in homes and in public, their fear that some malicious agent was responsible for their misfortunes. Southern Zimbabweans are not much different from people in other parts of the world. Similar observations have been made by anthropologists elsewhere. Yet Zimbabwe is an ideal setting to observe the dynamics of attributing responsibility for misfortune to some evil agent because of the rising number of individuals suffering from AIDS, which made the search for meaning more urgent and widespread. Generally, Zimbabweans did conclude that HIV/AIDS is widespread because an evil agent is at work.

During my anthropological fieldwork in 2001 and 2003, nearly everyone I met expressed their belief that the AIDS epidemic may be connected to the workings of an evildoer, frequently described as a sorcerer or a conspirator. I had established contact with one of the teachers at a primary school situated in the research site. She organized an AIDS Club for the pupils; they met once a week after school to socialize, to learn about HIV/AIDS, and to teach each other about the epidemic. The meeting I attended was an eye-opener for me regarding the prevalence of sorcery beliefs in Zimbabwean households. The group of students sang and danced. Translated into English, one song had the following refrain:

> The child is sick. They say the child is bewitched. It is bewitched by whom? They say by the neighbor.

Listening to this song, which they sang frequently at other occasions, I began suspecting that sorcery attributions for explaining misfortune in general and illness in particular were quite common. Why would children choose a song with that theme from their wide repertoire of songs? I concluded that it reflected a prevalence of sorcery beliefs within their families and households.

Another event enabled me to draw similar conclusions for conspiracy theories. I had taken part in a workshop on HIV/AIDS awareness in June 2001 in the small border town of Plumtree.[6] During the workshop, HIV/AIDS was clearly defined as a sexually transmitted disease and the individual's behavior cited as the ultimate factor responsible for acquiring the virus. This explanation, however, did not satisfy some participants of the workshop, who expressed suspicion that an evil-minded agent is responsible for the epidemic. The other participants of the workshop enthusiastically supported this argument, which then redirected the focus from how to prevent further infections to conspiracy suspicions of an insidious plot.

My impression that sorcery beliefs and conspiracy theories are a crucial element in people's discussions about the AIDS epidemic was later supported by ample evidence in my observations, in interviews, and in other sets of data. The fact that sorcery beliefs and conspiracy suspicions are common in Zimbabwe prompted me to investigate such explanations of the AIDS epidemic. Interpretation of these beliefs was supported by the long tradition in African Studies of investigating sorcery in Africa (see Douglas 1970:xxiii). Because sorcery beliefs and conspiracy theories are closely related, this tradition helped in the interpretation of the latter as well.

Though the arguments in this book are based on insights gained through my experiences in southern Zimbabwe, I found evidence that HIV/AIDS was interpreted similarly within social groups whose social, cultural, and historical background shares common features with that of southern Zimbabweans.

In Zimbabwe, making meaning through blame is a widespread phenomenon that exists far beyond AIDS discourse. Attributing blame to others for economic, political, and other misfortunes in Zimbabwe is a common practice and a familiar pattern of thought. This pattern is exemplified by a cartoon in the Bulawayo newspaper that comments on the rising costs of transport. When transport costs rose considerably during 2003, commuters blamed the bus operators, who in turn pointed the finger at private oil companies, who blamed the state-owned oil company, who then blamed the rising prices on the international oil industry. The common practice of finger-pointing when misfortune strikes is, for Zimbabweans, a well-established and familiar pattern within which interpretations of HIV/AIDS became anchored. Similar observations have been made elsewhere.[7] AIDS meanings, like other illness explanations, are highly context dependent and speak louder about society, culture, and values than they do about a disease.[8]

Clearly, individuals in any context use familiar patterns of making meaning when they encounter something new or unknown. But how, exactly, do specific explanations become attached to skyrocketing oil prices,

FUEL.....THE BLAME GAME.

Blaming dynamics. (*Harare Daily News,* September 1, 2003)

or to HIV/AIDS? Among the many strains of cultural theory concerning this issue, both within and outside anthropology, Moscovici's Social Representations Theory provides a useful tool for understanding the processes through which HIV/AIDS acquires meanings. Moscovici's use of the term *social representations* has its origin in Durkheim's (1974) concept of *collective representations*. However, while Durkheim was referring to characteristics of social thinking as distinct from individual thinking, which explains the integration and conservation of society, Moscovici (1976) applied it to questions of how things change in society.

Moscovici argues that within any culture there are points of tension and fracture around which new representations emerge. For instance, the sudden appearance of new and threatening phenomena, such as HIV/AIDS, can trigger the development of new representations (Duveen 2001b:8). Moscovici posits that these emerge when individuals engage in interaction with each other during the course of everyday conversations. Thus, Moscovici (2001b:146) even calls them a form of *Umgangsdenken* (everyday thought) associated with *Umgangssprache* (colloquial language). The result is a set of explanations originating in daily life in the course of inter-individual communications (Moscovici 1981:181).

Two specific processes are at work when people integrate new ideas: anchoring and objectification. Through anchoring, unfamiliar concepts are compared and interpreted in the light of phenomena generally accepted as common sense, as well as widely shared values, norms, and beliefs.[9] Blaming dynamics, sorcery beliefs, and conspiracy suspicions embody in Zimbabwe and elsewhere widely known thought patterns that assign responsibility to "others." These patterns of thought, within the social, political, and economic context, represent the familiar through which the new epidemic becomes anchored.

People understand novel experiences best by referring them to familiar domains (Fernandez 1986:25). Thus, emerging social representations owe much to convention and memories shared by members of a group, are likely to be fairly stable over time, and are not easily modified.[10] The anchored endproduct then becomes objectified into concrete mental content distinct from the original domain within which it first became anchored (Joffe 1999:94–95). These two mechanisms make the unfamiliar familiar, first by transferring it to a familiar sphere that allows people to compare and interpret it, and second by reproducing it among tangible things (Moscovici 2001b:42). Once social representations are created, they can be modified and reworked as they continue to evolve (Moscovici 2001b:27, 148, 158).

Moscovici, among others, did apply Social Representations Theory specifically to the evolution of the attribution of meanings to HIV/AIDS.[11] Their work exposes the manner in which traditional beliefs and familiar understandings attach themselves to the epidemic, evolve over time, and finally generate behavioral expectations in those who hold the views. I observed such processes occurring in the AIDS epidemic as I listened to people in Zimbabwe.

Social Representations Theory is useful in understanding such processes. In initial discussions about the epidemic, the disease was compared with familiar phenomena, the so-called anchoring. People identified correlations and distinctions with known diseases and epidemics such as historical epidemics, sexually transmitted diseases, sorcery-induced ailments, and negative health effects caused by others. I often heard statements such as "AIDS is like the Spanish influenza," or "AIDS is like syphilis," or "AIDS is like *isidliso*," an ailment related to sorcery that I describe in Chapter 5. People looked for the familiar in order to understand the unknown. Later in the attempt to comprehend the disease their statements changed because AIDS had developed meanings that did not depend on comparisons. Over time more people argued that "AIDS is sorcery," or "AIDS is a conspiracy!" The epidemic has become objectified.

Moscovici's theory may give the impression that the process of attributing meaning to new phenomena is a single and unidirectional societal event. My observations from Zimbabwe show that it is not as simple and straightforward as it seems. The temporal sequence from anchoring to objectification does not occur as a logical and singular event in society, though over the years perceptions about the epidemic moved from comparisons with familiar events to becoming increasingly objectified as they acquired an independent cognitive reality.

We have to keep in mind that this temporal sequence is not simply a societal tendency but strongly related to individuals and their engagement with the epidemic. I observed that while some people still compared AIDS with other familiar phenomena when searching for meanings for the disease, others already viewed the epidemic as a distinct phenomenon with its own meanings. The social and individual levels mingle and interact, influencing the processes by which the epidemic acquires meaning. And these meanings, as Moscovici points out, continue to evolve and change.

Another complicating issue is that the agency of individuals in familiarizing and objectifying HIV/AIDS depends on multiple factors beyond their control. I will show, for instance, how political interests and constellations, as well as the mass media, influence perceptions about the AIDS epidemic.

To sum up, Social Representations Theory is useful for understanding the general dynamics of how meanings become attributed to the AIDS epidemic. However, it does not focus on the specific factors, individuals' relations and agendas, or collective powers and prejudices, nor on historical and current political and economic realities. Only ethnography can uncover such specific factors. In this book I tried to tease out some of the factors that are relevant for understanding how Zimbabweans came to comprehend the epidemic.

Fellow anthropologists and others working in the field of HIV/AIDS awareness and prevention raise the question of the theoretical usefulness, as well as the applicability for practical means, of the study of sorcery beliefs and conspiracy theories attributed to the AIDS epidemic. Why, within the wide range of meanings ascribed to the AIDS epidemic, should we single out and study these two types of causal explanations? Is the study of sorcery and conspiracy theories not just contributing to the construction of an exotic "other" (e.g., Masquelier 2004:95; Pels 2003:14)? Sorcery beliefs and conspiracy theories were typically identified in traditional, non-Western societies, which were viewed as fundamentally distinct from industrialized Western societies. Does a focus on popular AIDS beliefs, which points the finger of blame to others, deviate attention from the sexual transmission of HIV? Would it not be more beneficial for public health programs curbing the spread of the AIDS epidemic to study local meanings attached to the disease that are more compatible with a definition of HIV/AIDS as a sexually transmitted disease (Green 1999:269–70)?

Though I share such concerns, I am convinced that a better understanding of sorcery beliefs and conspiracy theories, which became attached to the AIDS epidemic, yields theoretical insights into how people explain and react to health problems, and in turn benefits health programs. My focus on the two types of causal explanation is also supported by a renewed emphasis in anthropology on sorcery, and implicitly on the related category of conspiracy theories, after decades of their academic backstaging (Gusterson 2004:7).

Additional support comes from studies investigating the influence of illness beliefs on health-seeking behavior. There appears to be a cognitive link between people's beliefs about the etiology of disease and particular health-seeking behavior (Good 1987:15–18). Applied to the AIDS epidemic, this means that knowledge and attitudes toward HIV/AIDS, as well as the perceived causes of the HIV-infection, can influence the ways people approach preventing infection and seeking treatment and support. Numerous scholars follow this line of thought and argue that AIDS beliefs, including beliefs suspecting a deliberate plot behind the epidemic, must be addressed explicitly in culturally tailored AIDS prevention, treatment, and coping programs.[12] More specifically, conspiracy theories (and we can say the same for sorcery beliefs) exert tremendous influence on people's decisions to use means for preventing infection and to seek healthcare (Whetten-Goldstein and Nguyen 2002:180). It is necessary to understand such beliefs and their underlying rationales when designing HIV/AIDS healthcare programs.

The interpretation of HIV/AIDS as the result of either sorcery or a conspiracy has some obvious implications for HIV/AIDS awareness, for prevention of future infections, and for treatment of AIDS patients in Zimbabwe. Attention is diverted from sexual transmission of the disease to the doings of an evil agency that plots to harm one or more individuals. Those who hold the belief that some malicious "other" is behind the disease may not take the necessary precautions during sexual encounters because they see in AIDS the doings of some evil agent. For them it is more important to identify this agent than to protect themselves against infection. In other words, as people told me, if there is an evil force behind the disease, then neither prevention nor a cure will help. This agent will find another way to harm them!

A specific example relevant to healthcare is a widespread Zimbabwean rumor that a malicious agent inserted HIV into the lubricant of condoms. Those who believe this rumor distrust those who promote condoms and even suspect them of complicity with the unknown evil agent. In their interpretation, the use of condoms does not protect against HIV-infection but actually exposes the user to a direct risk! Such evidence in Zimbabwe and cross-culturally supports the widely held view that sorcery beliefs and conspiracy suspicions need to be considered when designing culturally appropriate HIV interventions and educational campaigns. Such campaigns would increase receptivity to information about preventing HIV-infection.

Chapter 1 briefly outlines the methods I used to study sorcery beliefs and conspiracy suspicions and underscores the difficulties connected to the study of the two types of causal explanations for the AIDS epidemic. These issues are not only pertinent to my Zimbabwean case study but also have cross-cultural applicability for the study of sorcery beliefs and conspiracy theories in this context.

Social Representation Theory encourages us to look for familiar patterns in order to understand meanings attributed to a new phenomenon. The societal context provides familiar patterns within which HIV/AIDS has acquired meaning. Thus, Chapter 2 describes the social, political, and economic context of the AIDS epidemic in Zimbabwe. Sorcery beliefs and conspiracy suspicions, part of the local *Weltanschauung* (worldview), are familiar patterns within which the epidemic became anchored. Chapter 3 presents aspects of the academic discussion on sorcery beliefs and compares them with what Zimbabweans told me. I then describe three specific Zimbabwean examples of sorcery practices that relate to local interpretations of why someone falls ill with AIDS-related symptoms: *undofa*, a witch's familiar (Chapter 4); *isidliso*, a sorcery poison used by women, and *ulunyoka*, a magical sorcery substance used by men (both described in Chapter 5). While these are specific to the Zimbabwean experience, I provide comparable phenomena from other societies and cultures indicating that the patterns apply cross-culturally.

Chapter 6 theorizes about conspiracy suspicions that relate to AIDS fears in Zimbabwe and other parts of the world. Subsequent chapters provide examples of particular conspiracy suspicions in rich ethnographic detail: conspiracy theories implicating health professionals (Chapter 7), and popular theories attributing blame to Westerners (Chapter 8). In both types of conspiracy suspicions, I identify certain patterns in the evolution of the beliefs that have cross-cultural relevance. Chapter 9 then identifies both types of beliefs in a Zimbabwean narrative that contains both sorcery beliefs and conspiracy suspicions, and concludes with the startling finding that people frequently shift their discourses from biomedical understandings of HIV transmission to social conjectures related to sorcery and conspiracy.

Chapter 10 concludes with an argument for the pragmatic approach of studying AIDS beliefs within the sorcery and conspiracy paradigms. In addition to offering theoretical insights, the chapter argues that understanding popular causal explanations is crucial to the success of programs aiming at preventing new HIV-infections and caring for those already suffering from AIDS.

Notes

1. Before 1980 Zimbabwe was called Southern Rhodesia, or simply Rhodesia, after Cecil Rhodes, the twentieth-century British explorer whose tomb is in the Matobo area near Bulawayo.

2. Theorists of sorcery frequently follow Evans-Pritchard's classic distinction between sorcery and witchcraft, which is discussed later in this book. As most of the evidence to which I refer is more closely related to sorcery than to witchcraft, I generally refer in this book to sorcery.

3. Key AIDS studies that draw a distinction between *disease* and *illness* include Brandt 1988; Cline and McKenzie 2000a, 2000b; Harter 1998; Herzlich 1995; Mann 1988:159; Romero-Daza 1994; Sindzingre 1995; Sontag 1990; Stansbury and Sierra 2004; Taylor 1990; Treichler 1989, 1999; Wolf 1996a, and 1996b.

4. See, for example, Feldman 1990:60; Grundlingh 1999:56; Joffe 1999:39; Niehaus and Jonssen 2005:180–81; Sabatier and Tinker 1988:105; and Schoepf 1995:37.

5. *Ndebele* refers in this book to the Zimbabwean Ndebele. Their language is generally

denoted by attaching a prefix, iSiNdebele. However, for the sake of clarity, I also use *Ndebele* to refer to the language of the Ndebele. Ndebele terms and concepts often closely resemble, or are even identical with, terms and concepts in the Zulu language. Due to this similarity, I do not make a distinction between the two languages.

6. This event is described in detail in Chapter 6.

7. See, for instance, Doka 1997:22; Douglas 1992:34; McGrath 1992; and Nelkin and Gilman 1991:41–53.

8. This argument has been convincingly brought forward, e.g., by Farmer 1988:80, 1994:806; Finerman and Bennett 1995:1; and Herzlich 1995:160.

9. See, for example, Hewstone 1989:208; Joffe 1996:174–77; Moscovici 1984, 2001b:30; and Moscovici and Hewstone 1983:105.

10. See, e.g., Joffe 1996:183, 1999:10, 105; and Moscovici 2001b:39.

11. See, for instance, Duveen 2001a:236–37; Joffe 1996:173–74, 1999:9–10; Moscovici 1987:154, 2001a:121; and Moscovici and Vignaux 2001:156.

12. See, for example, Aggleton et al. 1989; Bogart and Bird 2003a; Clark 1998; McGary, 1999; Ministry of Health and Child Welfare 1999; Guinan 1993; Jackson 2002; Klonoff and Landrine 1999; Nicoll et al. 1993; Smith 1999; Thomas and Quinn 1991; Washington 1998; and Woudenberg 1998. The same has been argued explicitly for AIDS conspiracies, e.g., by Bogart and Thorburn 2003b, 2005; Clark 1998; France 1998; McGary, 1999; Richardson 1997; Smith 1999; and Thomas and Quinn 1991.

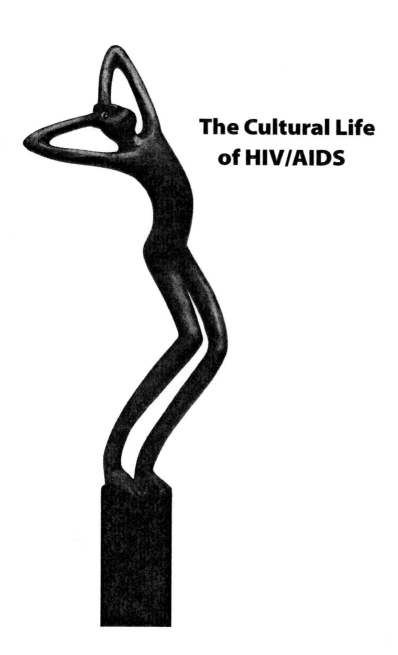

PART I

The Cultural Life
of HIV/AIDS

CHAPTER 1

Investigating Sorcery and Conspiracy

Despite my best efforts, quantifiable methods proved to be of limited usefulness for studying sorcery and conspiracy suspicions in Zimbabwe. The data underlying this Zimbabwean case study come from multiple sources, a common strategy in ethnographic fieldwork. I used various types of quantitative methods, including not only door-to-door interviews with a randomly selected sample of the target population but also several techniques of modern cognitive anthropology including free listing, pile sorting, and paired comparison, along with their concomitant analyses—but the results were disappointing. I will get to the reasons for this later.

In contrast, traditional ethnographic methods, such as different types of interviewing with individuals and groups selected by means of convenience sampling, as well as archival and mass media research, yielded an abundance of valuable data. In addition to both quantifiable and textual data, I have collected visual data in the form of photos, video-clips, newspaper cartoons, and even wood carvings of relevant themes by a local artist, Sheunesu Shumba.[1]

These types of data were collected through long-term participant observation, which is crucial to understanding sensitive issues such as sorcery beliefs and conspiracy theories (Herdt and Stoller 1990:17–18). Both types of belief are held in some degree of privacy or even secrecy, and individuals may express different views and convictions about them in public than they do in private. As Goffman observed, people shift between the normative, expected, and conventional "front-stage" behavior and the "back-stage" behavior that is hidden away from the public eye (Goffman 1959:22–30). Participant observation allows access to that backstage behavior because it can be done at various times for a large number of individuals in diverse social settings. It also allows a deep level of trust between the participant observer and the observed that is impossible to reach quickly, and it is essential for obtaining information about sensitive issues.

Beyond the choice of methods, the success of any research depends necessarily on the anthropologist and on the conditions under which he or she is conducting the research. As Schensul and colleagues have stated, the researcher is the "primary instrument of data collection" (Schensul et al. 1999:273–74). I conducted the case study in Zimbabwe in my double role as a Catholic priest and an anthropologist.[2]

Some colleagues in anthropology argue that the observing anthropologist is diametrically opposed to the intrusive missionary priest, thereby questioning the validity of some missionary findings. However, anthropologists have also pointed out that researchers are rarely neutral; they assume other roles depending on their gender, racial background, origin, and involvement (LeCompte et al. 1999:4–6). Being a priest is just one of these roles. Any role can introduce some errors by response effects (Bernard 2002:230), but it can also open up new avenues for collecting data. I believe that my priestly role at the research site was more an opportunity than a hindrance.

First of all, being a priest helped in establishing trust. As an example, when I was interviewing an elderly woman, she was upset that I as a "child" dared to ask her personal information! "Child" and "elder" are relative classifications that change depending on various characteristics of the two individuals and the circumstances of the encounter. In this case I was much younger than she, and thus in her eyes the child. Children do not ask elders personal questions.

When I later realized she was a Catholic, I went to her and introduced myself as a priest. Now the roles were changed; I was the elder and she the child. She had no problem responding to the questions I had asked her the day before. She may have even felt compelled to respond honestly to what the "father" asks from his "child." This illustrates how we anthropologists can actively draw on our various roles and so positively influence the interview process. My priestly role was often helpful in establishing trust between my informants and me.

Establishing a trust relationship is of crucial importance for investigating issues such as HIV/AIDS. The sensitive nature of AIDS-related issues imposes certain constraints on discourses that could compromise the validity of data and the success of a study (Leap 1991:285). The study of a sensitive issue such as HIV/AIDS necessitates a framework of trust and confidentiality (Abramson 1992:108). Being a priest placed me within such a framework, allowing me to collect valid data.

My priestly role, however, had only a limited positive impact on a related issue. In southern Africa, speaking about HIV/AIDS is a taboo-theme in the same way as sexual behavior, promiscuity, and prostitution are. These are not only taboo-themes because of their private or shameful nature. It is taboo to speak about these issues because of the cultural concept of "respect," called *inhlonipho* in Ndebele, which regulates much of social behavior, including who speaks in what manner about what topic with whom. *Inhlonipho* became a potential obstacle to communication across different genders, ages, and social statuses. To minimize *inhlonipho's* response effects to my age, gender, appearance, idiosyncrasy, and biases, including those potentially coming from my priestly role, I worked with several assistants of both genders, of varying ages, and of diverse ethnic and educational backgrounds.

Second, my role as a priest proved to be crucial within the context of the political and economic decline that Zimbabwe experienced during the years of my research. Any foreigner or person of European descent who conducted interviews was viewed with suspicion and mistrust by the political leadership. The members of the party in power, ZANU-PF, could have negatively intervened in my study. Actually, the officer in charge at the local police station near the research site gave me a stern warning to remain within the framework of strictly medical research—otherwise the police would arrest and deport me. For the duration of the study, church members protected me, their priest, when members of the party in power became suspicious about my movements.

Third, the priestly role helped me to respond to the immense suffering we witnessed every day without compromising the research. My assistants and I spent long hours discussing with informants the political and economic situation in the country, how HIV/AIDS affects their families and their neighbors, and how they cope with it. These discussions rarely remained calm and rational and frequently led to emotional expressions of pain and desperation. I was able to draw on my other identity, the priest, when I was asked to pray for people. Prayer offered some consolation in those dire circumstances.

I recall a visit in a household with four members: an elderly woman, her daughter, and her two grandchildren. The daughter spoke openly about the fact that she was dying of AIDS, soon to follow her husband who passed away a few months ago. She told me that her lastborn, an infant of about two years of age, who was in great pain, only skin and bones, was also HIV-positive. She and her child were looked after by her aged grandmother; her [the mother's] chief concern was what would happen to her firstborn, a boy of primary school age. She knew that he would soon be the only one left—with no money, living in an extended family stretched beyond its limits due to the harsh economic conditions in the country, and with hardly any support available from social welfare. She knew he could easily end up destitute. It was emotionally draining for us to be exposed to such extreme suffering.

It is difficult for researchers not to become emotionally involved with the suffering of their informants and respondents (Shelley 1992:79). Strong emotional involvement of the interviewer carries the potential risk of injecting one's feelings into the study, thus possibly biasing the data (Bernard 2002:219). I felt that my yearlong counseling experience as a priest helped me to separate my own emotional involvement from the information that I gained.

To sum up: The use of multiple types of methods, implementing the study with the help of assistants, and my dual role as a priest and an anthropologist, make me confident that both my data and my analyses are valid and a solid base from which to draw legitimate links between AIDS beliefs and beliefs related to sorcery and conspiracy.

Researching sorcery- and conspiracy-related beliefs pertinent to HIV/AIDS poses certain challenges that are particular to these types of beliefs. What follows relates mainly to the difficulty of studying sorcery beliefs but some of the arguments are also pertinent to the study of conspiracy theories.

The primary challenge is the difficulty in documenting both knowledge about sorcery and actual evidence of sorcery practices.[3] The lack of clear evidence about sorcery-related beliefs seems to be common cross-culturally. Generally, evidence is more accessible in societies where sorcery is not only used for nefarious ends but also, for instance, for protection. Most people with whom I talked had at least some belief in the existence of such practices, yet most claimed not to have any specific knowledge of what is needed for such practices, or how they are performed, or who could be approached about performing them. Although they hardly pinpointed actual evidence of such practices, they expressed belief in sorcery and their fear of it, debating the issue even as they feared possible consequences. In other words, people were greatly concerned about sorcery but had no firm evidence that anyone actually did anything, as the following quote from an interview[4] shows:

> We have never known someone who was bewitched. But sorcery exists and has to be taken seriously. However, we have never personally experienced it!

Some anthropologists interpret such statements of informants as an indication that sorcery beliefs are merely a way of speaking about a troubling social world. For them, sorcery simply explains misfortune, but most probably does not exist in reality.[5] However, the issue of the factual reality of sorcery (and, for that matter, of conspiracies) is not a focus of this book. I am more concerned with the reality of such beliefs in the minds of the people.

For those who hold beliefs in sorcery or conspiracies, these beliefs are perceived as real dangers that threaten the believer's well-being.

Consequently, the issue is not how we can find factual evidence of these secretive beliefs and practices, but how we can break through the veils of secrecy to gain access to the meanings and functions of sorcery beliefs and conspiracy suspicions. I found the following five issues important for explaining the reticence among my informants when asked about sorcery beliefs and conspiracy theories. These five issues complicated the study of such beliefs in Zimbabwe, and some of these issues are relevant for the study of sorcery beliefs and conspiracy theories elsewhere.

When discussing sorcery beliefs with Zimbabweans, I frequently observed that many carefully disassociated themselves from such beliefs and their suspected practice. The Zimbabwean interviewees most probably hesitated to articulate such information, fearing that I may think them to be sorcerers themselves. As elsewhere (e.g., Romberg 2003:209), in Zimbabwe no one wants to be suspected of being a sorcerer or of being implicated in sorcery practices. The headline of a report in a local Zimbabwean newspaper succinctly expresses such a sentiment, stating: "If you smell a witch, you are one yourself" (Wermter 2003). In other words, if you are able to identify a sorcerer by your knowledge of sorcery, you are potentially one yourself. After all, sorcerers are the ones who have expert knowledge on this issue (Niehaus 2001:12). When Ashforth (2000:50) asked a South African about the relation between sorcery and HIV/AIDS, the individual replied, laughing: "Don't ask me, I'm not a sorcerer. But I know they can do it."

Diviners and healers, who are the most likely to have knowledge of herbal and other potions used for sorcerous practices, were particularly defensive when asked about sorcery. Perhaps aware that they would be the prime suspects of sorcery practices, they adamantly denied any knowledge of them. They insisted that, although they are aware of such practices, they have no knowledge about how to prepare ingredients and perform rituals. In Zimbabwe, as elsewhere, people suspect that the powers and expertise of diviners and healers may be put to malign use. In many societies, diviners/curers are believed to have the power to control evil, and thus to be capable of using evil for nefarious purposes. Cross-culturally, the powers of diviners, healers, and shamans are frequently thought to be involved in benevolent as well as malevolent activities; thus diviners and healers are seen as ambiguous persons with the potential of being sorcerers.[6] Both can cure and inflict harm. Healing and sorcery are the "twin forces of white and black, of positive and negative" (Malinowski 1969:194). An Ndebele proverb similarly states that *inyanga ng-umthakathi*, literally meaning that the healer is a sorcerer, that the person who has medicine for healing also has medicine for harming.

The ambiguity of healers matches the ambiguity of what they use in their practices. In most Bantu languages, including Ndebele, there is no linguistic distinction between curative medicinals and substances believed to work in a destructive manner. Poisons, herbal mixtures, magical charms, and so on are all called in Zulu and Ndebele *umuthi*, and only the context and attributes define use and assign value. *Umuthi* is usually translated as "medicine" in English. However, the two terms are not synonymous, for *umuthi* can be used in attempts to destroy health as well as attempts to restore it. There is "medicine for healing," *umuthi wokwelapha*, and "medicine for killing," *umuthi wokubulala*. In other words, the healer's *umuthi* cures, while the sorcerer's *umuthi* kills (Ashforth 2005:139). *Umuthi* can be used for both purposes, depending on the intention of the user. The intrinsic efficacy of such "medicines" and powers remains latent and morally neutral until it is used by someone for either positive or negative purposes.[7]

Understandably, the people with whom I spoke, particularly the healers and diviners, wanted to make it clear that their *umuthi* is not used for malevolent purposes and that they lack knowledge of ways to prepare it for evil purposes.

A second methodological problem was that a Westerner was asking questions pertinent to sorcery. Residents in the township are aware that Europeans by and large discredit the efficacy of sorcery, at times even ridicule Zimbabwean ethnic groups for being superstitious and believing in such "ludicrous" practices. This widely held perception makes a discussion about sorcery between Zimbabweans and individuals of European descent challenging.[8] My informants downplayed such beliefs during interviews; they did not want to be judged superstitious. This does not mean that they did not believe in the existence and efficacy of sorcerous practices. They just did not want to share these beliefs with a Westerner. At times, people's fear of being thought superstitious coupled with their conviction that Westerners just do not understand the power of sorcery. I believe that people thought of me as totally incompetent to understand issues locally interpreted through the sorcery paradigm. Some gave the impression that they considered it a waste of time to talk with me about this issue. Studying conspiracy theories as a Westerner was also difficult. After all, most of the local AIDS conspiracy theories posit that Westerners are the masterminds behind the AIDS plot intended to harm them. I recall an incident during a focus group discussion. I had asked the participants to express their views on AIDS-related conspiracies. An elderly man was quite amused that I (being white, and a Westerner) asked this question. He bluntly told me that I would surely have better insights into conspiracies. After all, whites have created HIV in order "to get rid of all dark-skinned peoples!" The use of assistants successfully counteracted this potentially compromising issue.

A third methodological problem in studying sorcery is the fact that accusations pertaining to such practices are illegal in Zimbabwe, as they are in some other countries. The Witchcraft Suppression Act of 1899, though rarely applied, is still on the books[9] and anyone calling someone a sorcerer is potentially liable to a fine (Chavunduka 1986:46–47). The act warns diviners, when they are consulted by people asking them to identify the culprit suspected of being the cause for their misfortune, not to engage in such searches. In addition, the directives for members of the Zimbabwe National Healers' Association (ZINATHA) state that any healer involved in sorcery practices commits a crime. Such legislation and guidelines made it tricky to cast misfortune in terms of sorcery. Individuals convinced that sorcery is the source of their misfortune were unable to take appropriate steps for identifying sorcerers. Subsequently, the act drove the practice of sorcery underground and fostered secretive actions against assumed sorcerers (Chavunduka 2001:169; Mitchell 1960:197–201).[10]

Diviners and healers, instead of pointing at suspected sorcerers, emphasize the efficacy of powerful poisons and charms to counteract malign sorcery. People who suspect sorcery as the cause of their affliction are usually counseled quietly by a traditional diviner to consult a healer in order to obtain protective medicines (Auslander 1993:177). By and large accusations of sorcery are today restricted to the confidentiality of the extended family, where the authority structure within the family prevents individuals from contacting the local authorities. The following interview with a traditional healer supports such a conclusion:

> Healer: He was sick. He had a sickness of the heart.
> Interviewer: Was he bewitched?
> Healer: *Uhu*, can I say that someone was bewitched? Sorcery is a secret between me and my clients!

The matter of explaining misfortune through the workings of a sorcerer is essentially private. This complicates its study by outsiders.

This leads us to the selection of appropriate methods to study sorcery and conspiracy suspicions, the fourth methodological difficulty. I had to find a way that made it possible for people to disclose private and confidential information. The researcher's level of success in earning the trust of informants may explain some discrepancies and even contradictions in evidence across studies about the relation of sorcery beliefs to HIV/AIDS.[11] I believe the earning of trust depends partly upon the choice of the methodology used to collect information. I have observed a strong discrepancy between data derived through quick surveys and street interviews, and repeated interviewing in the homes of individuals based on trust and confidentiality. Information on sorcery collected by means of the survey questionnaire administered to a randomly selected sample of the target group, as well as information gathered through street interviews with respondents selected through convenience sampling, indicated a relatively low prevalence of sorcery beliefs and conspiracy suspicions in relation to HIV/AIDS. Information gained through repeated and long-term interviewing based on trust revealed that such beliefs and suspicions are strong in the minds of individuals and enthusiastically discussed in groups.

When randomly selected, the relationship with the prospective respondent was not necessarily based on trust, which suppressed people's willingness to admit sorcery beliefs. Frequently respondents courteously supplied me with the requested information, but I suspected that their responses did not match their own convictions. The issue of trust explains the discrepancy between the dearth of evidence of sorcery arguments in the surveys and ample evidence in the interviews. In other words, the validity of a study on sorcery beliefs and conspiracy theories heavily depends on the right selection of methods. Simple reliance on survey data could lead to an underestimation of the prevalence of sorcery beliefs. Therefore, most of my arguments are based on methods appropriate to the study of sorcery beliefs and conspiracy suspicions: trust-based interviews and other textual data.

A fifth methodological problem is that knowledge about and belief in sorcery as well as in conspiracy theories appears to be context-bound, changing, and evolving. Though everyone in Zimbabwe seemed to have one or another belief about the AIDS epidemic—after all, the AIDS epidemic is widespread and touches the lives of every family—the belief expressed during an interview may not be held constantly. Informants tended to respond differently depending on their particular involvement with HIV/AIDS. When asked about sorcery-related perceptions of HIV/AIDS, they may have discredited them; however, when a family member had full-blown AIDS, there appeared to be a greater likelihood that family members would blame the sickness on sorcery or a conspiracy. Similar observations were made elsewhere—that people tend to exhibit suspicions that sorcery is at work when they themselves suffer the consequences of some misfortune, while they would discredit such a view during better times (Ashforth 2005:124–26). Support for such an interpretation comes from my interviews with self-professed AIDS sufferers, from interviews with those whose bad health showed signs of AIDS-related illness, and from interviews with those who had an individual at home who exhibited such symptoms. These interviews show more references to sorcery than interviews with individuals who were not suffering directly from the effects of the AIDS epidemic.

To illustrate this argument, I present the case of a middle-aged man with AIDS who, after several unsuccessful attempts to get cured, finally concluded that his ailment was sorcery related. Several apparent AIDS sufferers and their families expressed similar arguments concerning the preternatural genesis of their ailment:

> These days many sicknesses are making our life difficult. When we are affected by one or another sickness, we usually go to the clinic where the nurses and doctors prescribe some pills. We take their medication and our condition improves, but after some time the disease comes back again. It starts again to trouble us! You have no idea if the ailment is AIDS or a condition caused by sorcery, or disgruntled ancestors—or if it is just a simple stomach ailment.
>
> When I went to the hospital they told me that they do not know what the cause of my suffering is. I spent about two weeks in the hospital and the doctor decided that perhaps my kidneys are the cause of the problem. He gave me some injections, but nothing helped; my condition did not improve. I saw another doctor who made some tests. He suggested that perhaps my spine has a problem and he gave me some pills. Then they said it could also be TB and gave me fourteen pills to take every day.
>
> Later we tried to get a cure through traditional means. The diviners and healers tried various treatments. But at the end they had to admit that they too are unable to help me. Then I went to the Prophets. Some of them killed a chicken and washed me with the blood of the chicken mixed with milk. This is their method of curing, but still nothing improved.
>
> I went to another prophet. He told me that there is something in the lower spine and that I should go to the experts to have it removed.[12] But I did not go!
>
> My mother told me that she saw a documentary on TV about a certain healer and encouraged me to see him. When I was ready to go to him my wife pleaded with me to let her come along. I did not want

to leave her behind. I was really troubled about what I should do with her.[13] So we went together and met this healer. He asked me "Friend, what is troubling you?" I told him that I am sick and that I have pain, that my feet are hot and that I sweat a lot, and that I am so weak that I go to bed around 5 o'clock. He told me that he would fix the problem for me the following day.

The next day he removed a black thing from me, which had thorns, and he also removed ten cents, and he said that these thorns were responsible for the pain that I had suffered for a long time, and that the ten cents were responsible for my feeling hot for a long time. He said that all is well now. I thought that I am finally cured. The healer gave me medicines to drink and of course I drank them! I continued to go to this healer whenever the ailment tried to haunt me again.

The only ailment that continued bothering me was diarrhea. When I drank water it came out again right away. I was afraid that after eating I would immediately soil myself. This was when I sent my wife to the clinic, telling her that perhaps the traditional medicines aren't helping me! Maybe it is better to go to the hospital. At the clinic I was given some pills. I took them and the diarrhea stopped. I could again go out of the house, but my feet were still weak.

Then the chest pain and the feet, the sweating and the pain began increasing again and once more I was not able to walk. I was quickly getting worse. The elders told me that I have been bewitched by some relative, and they pointed at my wife. The relatives then got together—you know, those troublesome ones. My father is one of them, the father who gave life to me. My mother was killed by him! You see how evil my father is. She became sick and could not walk any more; her legs were crippled and she could only be transported in a wheelbarrow.[14] She knew that he was using sorcery and killing people. He is the one causing all these troubles.

This individual narrating his illness and how he has been coping with it is a typical example of an AIDS sufferer who uses Western, traditional, and spiritual healthcare to get cured, sometimes simultaneously but more commonly consecutively. The lack of efficacy of the curing methods of a particular healthcare system often triggers a shift (Schoormann

CHIKWAMA   Tony Namate

Doubts that AIDS is a disease treatable through traditional means. (*Harare Daily News,* March 10, 2003)

2005:358–59). When a patient's health does not improve through Western healthcare, a traditional healer is consulted, and a presumptive cure is found through divination. When the patient is still not entirely cured through the use of traditional healthcare, doubt shadows the interpretation of the condition through the sorcery paradigm and the afflicted individual turns to some other type of healthcare for treatment. Such doubts are expressed in the accompanying cartoon, which was published in a local newspaper.

These shifts in the interpretation of illness are important when analyzing the evidence of sorcery beliefs. When I interviewed the above-mentioned patient, he was convinced that sorcery was the cause of his ailments. Had I spoken to him when he was still healthy, or still convinced of the efficacy of Western healthcare, he would probably have discredited such beliefs, despite prevailing suspicions within his family that his own father was a sorcerer. However, when Western healthcare strategies failed, the patient reverted once more to the sorcery beliefs. This example highlights the challenges faced by the ethnographer who wishes to investigate sorcery beliefs as well as conspiracy suspicions. Informants may express different views at different times and in different situations and health conditions. Only long-term research and participant observation allow the researcher to see a fuller picture and to identify valid associations between people's beliefs and the conditions shaping their lives.

Notes

1. He has been part of a group around Zephania Tshuma who engaged in wood carvings for years. Some of Shumba's works have been exhibited nationally and regionally. I met him in Nkulumane Township and visited his household once a week for three months. From our discussions about the AIDS epidemic, he carved for me a set of eighteen figures or groups of figures. Each carving represents either popular causal explanations of the epidemic, or local views on treating and curing the disease, or means for preventing further infections.

2. Other priest-anthropologists have extensively discussed the issue of being both a priest and an anthropological researcher, and the potential biases and advantages arising from this fact (e.g., de Rosny 1985; Tule 2004:1–23).

3. This issue was discussed, e.g., in Bowden 1987:184; Good 1987:94; Murray and Alvarez 1973:35; Obeyesekere 1975:4; Selby 1974:62; and Sidky 1997:62.

4. To illustrate my arguments and to show how complex people's theories of the origin of and infection with HIV are (containing diverse and even contradictory meanings and connotations), I quote extensively from fieldwork interviews. When translating them from the original Ndebele text, I opted for a free translation, removing redundant linguistic fillers and irrelevant lines of thought so common in casual conversations. To allow an easier reading, I also removed the standard "…" that indicates omissions from the original text. Subsequently, some of the quotes within this book substantially differ from the same quotes in my dissertation (Rödlach 2005). When I quote from a published text, I still use the conventional "…" to refer to omissions from the original text.

5. This argument has been put forward, for example, by Carneiro 1977:222; Ellen 1993:7–8; Honigmann 1947:229; Middleton 1967:59; Resner and Hartog 1970:375; and Sidky 1997:62. Some researchers were able to collect actual evidence of a popular inventory of evil rituals, e.g., Evans-Pritchard 1931:52; Galt 1991:738; and Lemert 1997:94. Even when evidence of concrete beliefs is unearthed, this merely shows that some detailed knowledge about sorcery practices exists and does not prove that these practices were really followed.

6. Key studies discussing this argument are Ashforth 2005:7; Behringer 2004:45; Galt 1991:742; Leiban 1967:27; Loeb 1929:79-80; Park 1934:110; Pollock 1996:330; Pócs 1999:107; Siegel 2003:146; Stephen 1987b:73-74; Sweet 2003:161; and Whitehead 2002:203.

7. This has been argued, e.g., by Bloomhill 1962:30; Harwood 1970:71–74; and Turner 1968:14. For more detailed discussions on the ambiguous meaning of *umuthi* in the context of southern African languages see, for example, du Toit 1985:166 and Ngubane 1976:319.

8. Comparable observations were made, e.g., by Ashforth 2005:69; Conco 1979:74; and Kiernan 1977:3.

9. It has been argued by some that this law was apparently repealed in 1981 with the introduction of the Traditional Medical Practitioner's Act (e.g., Mutizwa-Mangiza 1999:4) while others hold that the act is still in use (e.g., Chavunduka 1982:2–4). Recent examples of trials on grounds arising from the act are known in Zimbabwe (Simmons 2002:304). The core problem of the act is that it conflates divination and some healing practices with sorcery, though divination and healing practices have a much wider application. The Act of 1981 introduces this distinction, but this has not yet entered common knowledge (e.g., Anonymous 1997b).

10. Paradoxically, there is evidence that witch hunts are happening with little or no interference by the law (for instance, the witch-cleansing hunts by Mabhebha observed by me several years ago in a rural area in southern Zimbabwe). Witch hunts have been reported elsewhere, e.g., by Yamba 1997.

11. While some scholars argue that in South Africa popular understandings of HIV/AIDS can be framed within the familiar sorcery paradigm (e.g., Ashforth 2001a:1; Marcus 2002:90), others discovered that discourses on HIV/AIDS in South Africa were seldom located within the sorcery paradigm (e.g., Niehaus and Jonssen 2005:180–81). Some variation in the evidence of such beliefs in different social settings is expected. Belief systems, including sorcery and conspiracy beliefs, depend on the societal and cultural context within which they were generated. They can wax and wane with changing societal and cultural conditions (Ardener 1970; Romanucci-Ross 1977). However, contradictory findings in comparable settings are somewhat startling and need explanation.

12. The belief that sorcerers are able to place various items into the body of the victim, and that they need to be removed by healers, is quite common. My interviews, as well as reports in the mass media, give ample evidence for such beliefs and practices (e.g., Anonymous 1991h).

13. He did not explain why he was concerned that his wife stay behind. The most probable reason is that she would have been accused of neglecting him. If something had happened to him on the way, she would have been the first one suspected of using sorcery.

14. Wheelbarrows are sometimes used in the townships in the absence of wheelchairs to transport sick people who are unable to walk.

CHAPTER 2

HIV/AIDS as Personal Experience

When people expressed their suspicions to me that someone was instrumental in the spread of HIV/AIDS, a sorcerer or a conspirator, they frequently referred to historic and current events or conditions that negatively shaped the course of the country's fate and individuals' lives. This became particularly apparent when they discussed AIDS conspiracy theories. To understand why, we need to know more about the conditions at the research site, the specifics of the Zimbabwean AIDS epidemic, and the politico-economic climate in the country. These are familiar configurations within which HIV/AIDS became established. I believe the Zimbabwean case study likely exemplifies processes that are occurring globally in a diversity of settings.

The case study was conducted in a township in Bulawayo, the second largest city in Zimbabwe, whose history[1] can be traced back to precolonial times. It was the site of the capital of the Ndebele kingdom with the same name. In the second half of the nineteenth century, European traders, missionaries, and administrators extended their sphere of influence in the

Ndebele kingdom, which led to several violent clashes with the Ndebele warriors. Toward the end of the 1893 Ndebele War, king Lobengula set fire to his capital and fled northward. British forces occupied the site immediately. European settlement began right away, resulting in the official founding of the city in 1894. The new European town grew rapidly and became the major link between South Africa and Salisbury—now Harare, and the colony's economic center. The fall of the Ndebele kingdom, the establishment of European rule, and the acquisition of the land is a legacy prevailing in political discourses and influencing even interpretations of HIV/AIDS presented in this book.

From 1960 onward nationalist politics became an increasingly powerful force in Bulawayo. In 1965 Zimbabwe unilaterally declared its independence from Great Britain, claiming itself a constitutional monarchy under the sovereign of England, and determined to preserve the power and influence of the European settlers in the country. During the 1960s and 1970s the political struggle for majority rule[2] intensified. In 1980, when majority rule was finally established, the population in the city was estimated to be more than 400,000. The years from 1983 to 1987 were unsettling for Bulawayo due to armed conflict in the southern part of Zimbabwe, with violent responses by the national government targeting the minority ethnic groups in the south, particularly the Ndebele.

In recent years, the significance of the city has been overshadowed by the growth of the country's capital, Harare. Many major companies transferred their headquarters out of Bulawayo, partly owing to recurring water shortages in the city. The political turmoil of recent years caused economic decline and many firms closed. Nevertheless, despite having lost much of its economic vigor and its political relevance, the population of Bulawayo is still growing (Dlodlo 2003:7).

The history of Bulawayo and its surrounding areas has resulted in a population of diverse ethnic groups—chiefly the Rozwi, Nambya, Venda, Kalanga, Ndebele, Tonga, and Europeans. In addition, with the construction of the railways and ensuing industrialization, large numbers of Malawians, Zambians, and Mozambicans migrated to Bulawayo. The various subgroups of the Shona cluster that represents the majority of Zimbabweans have been migrating to the city throughout the last decades and still continue to do so.

Bulawayo's ethnic composition becomes even more convoluted through frequent patterns of intermarriage between individuals of different ethnic groups, not to mention those second- and third-generation Bulawayo residents who may claim a particular ethnic identity but who were born and raised in the city and speak the city's vernacular, Ndebele. Bulawayo's ethnic *potpourri* is not particularly different from that of other world cities. The interaction of its ethnic groups is relevant for us, however. Individuals of diverse ethnic backgrounds have been mingling their views, including inherited beliefs and practices about sorcery—and, by extension, about conspiracies—resulting in widely shared hybrid beliefs with a common structure, a phenomenon found all over the world (Ashforth 2002:126–27). This process was made relatively easy through an already-existing commonality of ideas and practices about sorcery and conspiracies.

The principle of segregating and housing African dwellers in their own quarters, the so-called townships or locations, was common in pre-independent southern African countries. These townships were historically characterized by overcrowded basic housing, contrasting with the well-groomed towns and large bungalows of the white suburbs. In this regard, Bulawayo has been no exception.[3] After majority rule was achieved, the racially motivated division of the city was abandoned. Instead of a racial division, a mainly economic division remained: the middle-to-high income group lives in the relatively well-maintained, low-density Eastern Suburbs, while the bulk of resident low-income earners live in the high-density, poorly maintained Western Suburbs.

I conducted my research in the poor western suburb of Nkulumane Township in Bulawayo. Compared with other townships of the city, it is relatively new; the oldest sections of this township were constructed in the late 1970s. In 2003 the population was around 95,000. Nkulumane is subdivided into four municipal wards. I selected Ward 20 for the study, a residential area typical for urban high-density townships with a population of around 28,000 residents. Wards are significant to residents because the boundaries determine the voting limits of the area. Residents of a ward vote to elect a municipal counselor who supervises the area's events and organizations, for instance, the Ward AIDS Action Committee. Ward 20, unlike some other wards, even instituted a communal court dealing with minor conflicts among residents. Despite positive intentions, most of these organizations are not contributing much to the well-being of the ward residents. When I conducted the research, these ward groups were dominated by members of the ruling party, the ZANU-PF, and functioned to strengthen the position of the government. Their position in the township had some influence on the evolution of conspiracy theories. They promoted the government's claim that powerful "others" have been inflicting harm on Zimbabweans and still intend to do so. One of the evil agents' means to reach this goal is the AIDS epidemic.

At the research site, as elsewhere in Zimbabwe, suffering of individuals, families, and households due to the AIDS epidemic is evident. The progression of the disease at the research site matches the disease's evolution in the country.[4] The first AIDS cases were seen in Zimbabwe in 1983, but the problem was not recognized until 1985. There has been a steady increase in the number of AIDS cases reported and in the estimates of existing HIV-infection. HIV/AIDS prevalence was estimated for 2003 at around a quarter of the adult population (ages 15 to 49), with some 1.8 million Zimbabweans estimated to be living with HIV. Very mobile social groups have considerably higher numbers. There is some evidence that the number of new HIV infections is declining, and it is thought to be associated with behavioral change.

The total number of AIDS-related deaths during 2003 was projected to reach more than 170,000, close to 500 each day, with around 70% in the 15 to 39 age group. In 2004 HIV/AIDS was projected to take the lives of over 30% of the Zimbabwean population in the following decade. Mainly as a result of HIV/AIDS, Zimbabwe's life expectancy at birth has declined from its peak of over 60 years in 1985 to around 45 years in 2001, and it is projected to decrease further in the coming years. That people are aware of this is reflected in the accompanying cartoon (page 39) from a local newspaper. Bulawayo, the city where I conducted the study, follows the nationwide trend.

The shockingly high death rate has resulted in a high awareness of the epidemic among Zimbabweans and residents at the research site.

SAMSON   Noah Pomo

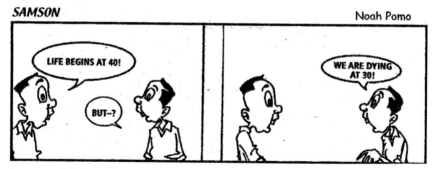

Awareness of declining life expectancies. *(Harare Daily News,* January 18, 2003)

More than half of the participants in our survey told us that they personally know many who exhibited symptoms possibly related to HIV/AIDS.
An overwhelmingly high number admitted one or more AIDS-deaths in
the extended family. The presence of HIV/AIDS in their lives translated
to frequent and emotional conversations and discussions about the epidemic, mainly with their peers at work or school but also with family
members. A local Bulawayo-based group has composed a song with the
title *Ingculaza,* a term that denotes HIV/AIDS (Ramadu 2001). Its refrain
highlights the pain and suffering caused by the epidemic and poses the
question asked by many informants, namely, how to respond to the epidemic. Many residents first looked to the government, arguing that it is
the government's duty to establish programs to curb the spread of the
epidemic.

In 1987 the Ministry of Health and Child Welfare established the National AIDS Control Program. Little was accomplished due to the lack of
funding and manpower as well as the secrecy surrounding the epidemic.[5]
From 1990 the government took a more open approach, supplied more
funding, and attempted better coordination of programs. In 2000 the government set up an AIDS levy, a 3% surcharge on income and corporate
tax, becoming the first nation to introduce a tax specifically designed to
raise money for awareness campaigns, testing expenses, and organizational costs, as well as antiretroviral (ARV) drugs. However, large amounts of
funds raised through the levy were lost due to bureaucracy, lack of ac-
counting, and inefficient organizational structures. Allegations were widespread that funds collected through the levy were misappropriated by the

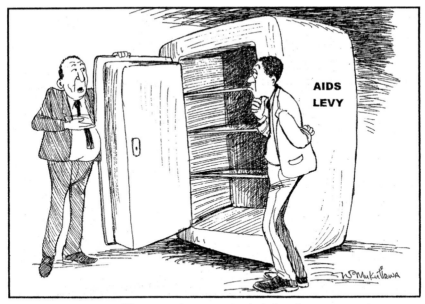

"The money is supposed to be in here."

Suspicions of misappropriation of the AIDS levy. (*Harare Daily News,* April 26, 2003.)

National AIDS Council and its subsidiaries.[6] This too is reflected in a cartoon that was published in a local newspaper (above). Not surprisingly, Zimbabweans lacked confidence in government support. A local newspaper quoted a widow:

> It is unacceptable for the government to watch at a distance thousands of its people starving and nothing is done. Most people are dying of HIV/AIDS-related illnesses that are hastened by the shortage of drugs. (Nkomo 2003b)

This perception matches evidence from Ward 20. For example, nearly half of all respondents in the random sample of my research said they believed HIV/AIDS spread so rapidly in Zimbabwe because the AIDS levy was misappropriated by politicians and civil servants. One township resident told me:

The government is not able to provide treatment for AIDS sufferers because of corruption, despite the availability of treatment on the market; the government diverts funds meant for AIDS-sufferers and politicians dine in fancy hotels using the funds. Those who are supposed to benefit from the funds are suffering at home without any help.

Respondents knew that various nongovernmental organizations (NGOs) working in the field of AIDS awareness and prevention had established a presence in the city and township but by and large, they thought, the NGOs failed to have a positive impact on peoples' lives. Their funds did not reach the needy:

There are a lot of AIDS organizations formed for the benefit of AIDS-sufferers, but people employed by them drive posh cars and the sufferers starve at home. Monies set aside for AIDS-sufferers do not benefit AIDS-sufferers, but enrich the AIDS agencies and their coordinators, while the suffering of people increases.

In addition, residents resented the wealthy Western nations, whose pharmaceutical companies refuse to sell the drugs to Zimbabwe at affordable prices. One example follows:

The Western countries develop new drugs but sell them at a very high price knowing that Zimbabwe is a poor country. I am unable to buy drugs for such high prices. How much more an AIDS patient is unable to buy the medicine that is needed. The AIDS patients need many medicines because they cough and have diarrhea, need special food, and many more things.

Other studies corroborate the finding that people feel abandoned by the government, NGOs, and the international community. The most reliable sources for any support for AIDS sufferers and their families were neither government nor NGOs but the extended family and, to a lesser degree, neighbors and other support groups.[7]

Hardships due to the AIDS epidemic were aggravated by the economic and political realities. Once regarded as the emerging star of postcolonial Africa, Zimbabwe was during my fieldwork a nation on the brink of political collapse (International Crisis Group 2003:1; Price-Smith and Daly 2004:9). Many people publicly expressed their disappointment, as did a Zimbabwean poet who described his country as an extraordinary flower, surpassing the beauty of other flowers, but now being destroyed by the government (Revilo 2003). Due to this common perception, the government's popularity was rapidly declining (Moyo and Makumbe 2000a, 2000b). The government responded to the loss of support among the electorate by becoming increasingly totalitarian and oppressive, attempting to silence any opposition to their policies by violent means. Obviously, this situation causes people to exercise great care about what they say (Chikwanha et al. 2004:24). My informants expressed fear that if the Central Intelligence Office (the national secret police) got hold of their statements, they may be "meeting a black dog." This popular sarcastic saying goes back to the death of the respected Bulawayo M.P., Sidney Malunga. His driver claimed the car had swerved because he tried to avoid running over a black dog. Rumor had it that the accident was a politically motivated assassination, a frequently used tool of the government to silence critical opposition.[8] Peoples' perceptions of this climate of intimidation and spying are reflected in the accompanying cartoon (top of page 43). If people felt inhibited about free expression, and if they therefore censored their public utterances, then my research data may not be reliable. Having established trust with respondents, however, I am confident that I counteracted this issue. I also showed people that their identity cannot be traced through my notes. In one incident, I deleted all references to individuals in my written notebook in the presence of a man afraid that his comments could become public.

Such fears are grounded in recent historical experiences of people in southern Zimbabwe. Soon after assuming power in 1980, the government was responsible for the killing and torture of thousands of unarmed civilians from 1983 to 1987 in the country's southern provinces, the stronghold of its main political rival (Zimbabwe Human Rights NGO Forum 2001b:2). The most dramatic manifestation of violence, intimidation, and intolerance of dissent was in the mid-1980s, when the govern-

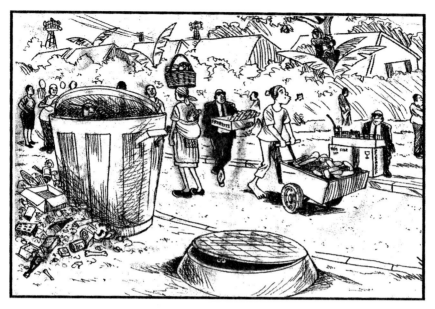

Zimbabwean secret police spying on the country's citizens. *(Harare Daily News,* March 18, 2003)

ment created the Fifth Brigade, notoriously known as the *Gukurahundi* (in Shona, "the early spring rain that washes away the chaff") to fight dissidents in the Matabeleland and Midlands provinces. Their actions were, as Rotberg (2002:228) states, "ethnic cleansing at its worst." Their reign of terror is responsible for the murder and disappearance of between 20,000 and 30,000 Zimbabweans, for aggravating ethnic tensions, and for generating a popular conviction that political freedom of expression was not permissible in Zimbabwe. A Unity Accord was signed in 1987 by the warring parties that effectively ended the conflict. The accord was succeeded by a presidential amnesty, which pardoned all dissidents, and the Clemency Order of 1990, pardoning all state security forces for atrocities committed by them.[9] Government supporters continued to intimidate residents in Bulawayo, threatening them with a return of the *Gukurahundi* if they do not support the government. Army helicopters hovering at low altitude over the townships during labor strikes in 2003 triggered fears among many of my informants that the government was about to unleash its force again. One informant told me that "the war has started now."

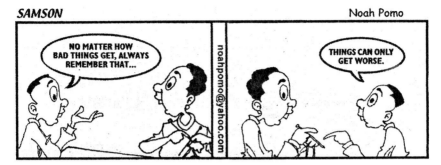

Awareness of bleak future. *(Harare Daily News,* June 11, 2003)

Further, the government showed overt disrespect for the rule of law, promulgating acts that safeguarded its powers and limited the freedom of expression and assembly.[10] My survey questionnaire tapped into responses of residents to these challenging political conditions. The overwhelming majority of respondents viewed the situation in Zimbabwe negatively, often adding during interviews that *ifuture kayikho* ("there is no future") and at times even arguing that things could only get worse. Such perceptions are reflected in the accompanying cartoon from a local newspaper (above). Some said that today *kuyafanana ukufa lokuphila* ("life and death are the same"), and added that in a few years we all will be dead because of civil war, or from hunger.

Although informants during interviews lamented the failure of the current administration to govern, many were more concerned with the dire economic issues affecting their lives.[11] Since the late 1990s the country has experienced grave economic hardship, becoming one of Africa's smallest and least productive economies, with persistent shortages of basic commodities. A lawless and chaotic land acquisition led to a drastic decline in food production. Rallying support among the shrinking number of its supporters, the government embarked on a massive campaign to acquire commercial farmland, promising to resettle landless citizens. With scarcely any farm able to operate undisturbed, agricultural production—including the harvest of export-oriented crops—was drastically reduced during recent years. The subsequent shortage of foreign currency resulted in a further contraction of the economy.

The Consumer Council of Zimbabwe in September 2004 pegged unemployment at 70% nationwide. A comparably high unemployment was also evident in Nkulumane during my fieldwork. Analysts argue that in 2003 at least 90% of Zimbabweans lived below the poverty datum line, while more than 50% were below the food datum line. Bulawayo followed the national trend, and the City Health Department even reported some deaths due to starvation. An Ndebele proverb, often heard in the township, describes such conditions: "The cat sleeps in the fireplace," meaning that there is nothing to be cooked in the house and the fireplace is so cold that the cat can sleep there. Most residents at the research site felt the brunt of the economic decline and were hardly able to make ends meet.

The deplorable economic conditions in Zimbabwe had a disastrous impact on the national health. Only a decade ago, Zimbabwe's public health system was above those of most nations of sub-Saharan Africa. But in 2003 shortages of even the most basic drugs, temporary unavailability of food, and breakdown of equipment were common in hospitals. When healthcare was available, it was unaffordable for most township residents. People reported hesitating to consult a doctor or a clinic. Many residents just stayed home when they were sick, hoping that their condition would not warrant treatment. The following quote from Nkulumane points up this situation:

> In the radio they speak that there are pills which really help when you have AIDS, but who can buy them? We don't have even enough food to strengthen our body. We can't even afford to see the doctor at the clinic. Everyone needs money to see the doctor, to get a prescription, and to buy medicine.

This finding is supported by other studies that report that the number of sick people not seeking medical attention rose dramatically over the last years due to healthcare costs.[12] This is reflected in the accompanying cartoon from a local daily newspaper (page 46). Particularly hard hit were individuals suffering from AIDS-related ailments. Antiretroviral

CHIKWAMA   Tony Namate

Difficulty of access to healthcare. *(Harare Daily News,* January 6, 2003)

drugs were virtually unavailable. Despite repeated announcements that the government plans to import them, Zimbabwe has been the country in southern Africa with the lowest access to AIDS drugs.[13] Respondents sometimes lamented that:

> When you have AIDS, the doctors in the hospital just give you pain-killers.

Some interviewees told me that they are only able to obtain ARV drugs through relatives working outside the country, particularly overseas, who have both the funds for purchasing and access to such medication. Not surprisingly, in Zimbabwe, as in other African countries, popular perception made a link between HIV, economic policies, and poverty, which was expressed through the assertion that the acronym *AIDS* stands for *"acute income* deficiency syndrome."[14] A cartoon in a local newspaper explicitly refers to this perception (page 47). Similar sentiments were frequently expressed by residents during interviews, but, due to the climate of political intimidation, most people hesitated to express their dissatisfaction directly.

Despite people's reluctance to speak about such conditions, the crisis-driven historical, political, and economic climate within which HIV/ AIDS arose in Zimbabwe has had substantial influence on the meanings attached to the epidemic. HIV/AIDS became anchored in the historical and contemporary experience of Zimbabweans. Sorcery and conspiracy

CHIKWAMA   Tony Namate

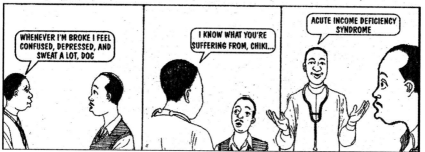

AIDS related to economic distress. *(Harare Daily News,* December 7, 2002)

fears about the AIDS epidemic were triggered by such circumstances. This argument is laid out in the following chapters and presents a pattern for the way the AIDS epidemic acquired meaning elsewhere.

Notes

1. Excellent sources for the history of southern African cities and Bulawayo are, e.g., Azevedo 1989; Catholic Commission for Justice and Peace and Legal Resources Foundation 1999; Dube 1994; Kaarsholm 1994; Pasteur 1994; Ransford 1968; and Rasmussen and Rubert 1990.

2. The phrase *majority rule* is usually associated with the South African struggle to end white domination by allowing every adult individual to vote, thus giving the majority (instead of a white minority) a say in who governs. I generally apply this phrase to Zimbabwe to denote the event in 1980 that ended white supremacy and rule. Generally this event is referred to in Zimbabwe as "independence." National political independence, however, should not be equated with individual political freedom. The current oppressive regime and the dehumanizing economic conditions render the term *freedom* inapplicable to the present situation.

3. More detailed information on townships in southern Africa in general and Bulawayo in particular can be found, e.g., in Ashton 1994; Connelly 1983; Epstein 1967; Government Town Planning Office 1951; Gussman 1952; Kaarsholm 1994; Hasler 1989; Knight 1994; Ndubiwa 1972, 1974; Patel 1988; Rödlach 2005; and Wekwete 1987.

4. The information in this and the following two paragraphs was drawn from my research data and the following sources: Dlodlo 2002, 2003; Gregson et al. 2006; Jelmsa et al. 2003; Msipa 2004; Price-Smith and Daly 2004; Robinson and

Marindo 1999; Ross et al. 2003; Sibanda 2000; and UNAIDS and World Health Organization 2004.

5. More information on factors contributing to the failure of the early programs are, e.g., in Bassett and Mhloyi 1991; Jackson and Mhambi 1992; Meursing and Sibindi 1999; Palmiere and Grant 2001; Ross et al. 2003; Schmitt 1999; Webb 1997; and Whiteside 1993.

6. The controversy over the misuse of the fund is reported, e.g., by Anonymous 2003a, 2003e; Chikuhwa 2004:176; National AIDS Council 2003; Mutemi 2003; Mutasa 2003b; and Price-Smith and Daly 2004:34.

7. The issue is well documented by Grant and Palmiere 2003:233; Jackson and Mhambi 1994:34; Palmiere 2000:167; and Palmiere and Grant 2001:168.

8. This argument has been extensively discussed, e.g., by Anand et al. 2004:6; Cheater 2001:25; Chikuhwa 2004:120–29; Catholic Commission for Justice and Peace 2000:96–97; Games 2002:11; Kagoro 2003:10–11; Makumbe and Compagnon 2000:245, 261; Price-Smith and Daly 2004:25; Raftopoulos 2001:24; and Zimbabwe Human Rights NGO Forum 2001a:14, 2001b:2, 2002:5, 2003:10.

9. See, for example, Kagoro 2003:6; Mair and Sithole 2002:23; Catholic Commission for Justice and Peace 2000:105; and Catholic Commission for Justice and Peace and Legal Resources Foundation 1999:60.

10. This has been well-documented, e.g., by Anand et al. 2004:6–7; Chikuhwa 2004:132; MacLean 2002:520; Mair and Sithole 2002:2–6; Meldrum 2005; Price-Smith and Daly 2004:25; Saller 2004:65–95; and Zimbabwe Human Rights NGO Forum 2003:12.

11. Regarding the economic conditions in Zimbabwe and Bulawayo see, e.g., Anonymous 2003b; Chikuhwa 2004; Catholic Commission for Justice and Peace 2000; Crisis in Zimbabwe Coalition 2003; Dube 2003b; Games 2002; International Crisis Group 2003; Msipa 2004; Mujokoro 2003; Nkomo 2003a; Price-Smith and Daly 2004; and Rotberg 2002.

12. This startling finding has been documented also, e.g., by Bassett et al. 1997; Dhliwayo 2001; Mwanza 1999; Tembo and Kupe 2002; and Winston and Patel 1995.

13. See, for example, Anonymous 2003f, 2003c, 2004; Hansen et al. 2000:438; Jackson et al. 1999:23; Johwa 2004; Mupedziswa 1998:124; Mutasa 2003a, 2003c; Nowak and Kähkönen 2004:37; Ross et al. 2003:31; and Stamps 1999:4710.

14. This association has been documented elsewhere, e.g., in Schoepf 1995:37–38; Setel 1999:145–46; and van den Borne 2005: 58–59.

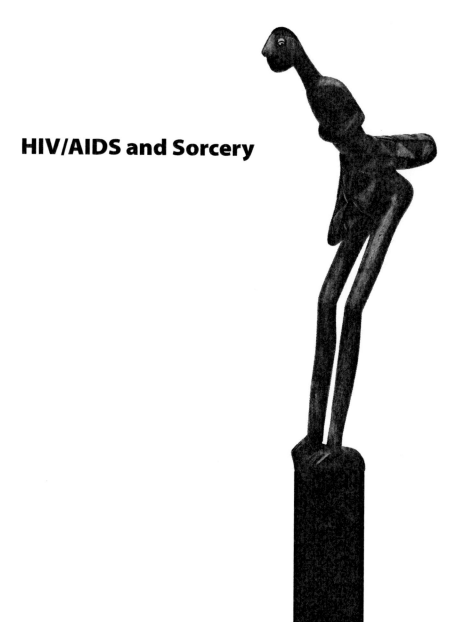

PART II

HIV/AIDS and Sorcery

CHAPTER 3

The Sorcery Paradigm

The AIDS epidemic has become anchored not only in the historic and contemporary experience of Zimbabweans but also in their shared thought patterns. A familiar pattern is the suspicion of sorcery. Because sorcery beliefs have worldwide distribution, they are crucial in understanding perceptions of and reactions to misfortune, illness, and death.[1] Diseases tend to elicit sorcery beliefs, which may play a minor role in some societies, but are inseparable from virtually all systems of disease etiology.[2] In regions inundated by HIV/AIDS, we can expect that people will refer to sorcery beliefs as they try to understand the epidemic. My Zimbabwean study illustrates this dynamic.

Though sorcery and related terms are labels for comparable phenomena, they differ radically within a society, and from society to society.[3] Depending on community practices, accusations may be made within a local group or between members of different communities. Sorcery may be tied mainly to socially condemned practices or a society may find legitimate uses of sorcery. Thus, universally acceptable definitions of sorcery—the "aggressive use of supernatural techniques that are based on an empirically non-demonstrable causation" (Walker 1989:3), or the "illicit use of extraordinary or supernatural power to cause harm" (Darling 1999:734)—necessarily remain problematic.

We need to arrive at a broader understanding of such phenomena without destroying their specificity (Forth 1993:116–17; Kapferer 1997:9–11). The varying interpretations by scholars reflect the diversity of sorcery beliefs, their meanings, and their functions. I cite here the interpretations relevant for my Zimbabwean case study but they reflect comparable interpretations of HIV/AIDS elsewhere.

Perhaps the most influential interpretation in the early research of sorcery is Evans-Pritchard's (1931:28; 1976b:1) distinction between inborn *witchcraft* and learned *sorcery*. While some scholars argue that this distinction cannot explain comparable beliefs among some ethnic groups, others hold that some sort of distinction between an innate capacity and a learned skill is evident among ethnic groups across the world. At times such a distinction is made within a society, but it is not likely to be made through use of distinct linguistic terms.[4]

My own observations in Zimbabwe support the latter argument. There is some distinction made between an innate and a learned capability but both a witch and a sorcerer are, for the Ndebele, an *umthakathi*! In conversation it becomes evident what the speakers refer to: if the evil-doer has a deep-rooted and persistent maliciousness, and comes from a family with a history of inflicting harm, then the appropriate English term for this person would be *witch*. In contrast, if the evil-doer is generally perceived to be an acceptable member of society and from a reputable family, then the person is called a *sorcerer*.

Most people I interviewed were less concerned with subtle distinctions and more interested in the means by which malicious humans inflict harm on others. How could, or would, these evil persons trigger misfortune? People I spoke with referred to three broad types of sorcery techniques:

1. Use of substances and poisons that become operational when the victim comes in touch with them; they are either put in victims' food or drink, placed in their path, or inserted into their bodies by other means.

2. Use of substances that operate magically without requiring physical contact.
3. Use of familiars that are sent to victims to cause misfortune.

The particular usages that I heard about in Zimbabwe are:

1. The *isidliso* poison becomes operational in the body of the victim.
2. The *ulunyoka* substances require some sort of physical contact with the victim, but operate mainly in a magical way.
3. The *undofa* is a familiar through which the sorcerer harms his or her victim.

I discuss *ondofa* in Chapter 4 (*ondofa* is the plural of *undofa*), and *isidliso* and *ulunyoka* in Chapter 5.

Anthropologists observed that, whenever misfortune is experienced, sufferers ask a series of questions (Mary Aquina 1968:47). Initially they ask how it happened, which probes the physical cause. The next two questions ask why it happened to this particular person and why at this particular time. These questions arise when there is seemingly unmerited suffering. Residents in Nkulumane asked the same questions, pondering why individuals have AIDS who did not appear to deserve it. AIDS victims were not always promiscuous individuals who, according to common perception, were likely to have contracted HIV. Observers viewed the HIV infection of those who were believed to have abstained from sex before marriage and been faithful to their spouses as unmerited, and therefore suspicious. Reference to sorcery explained this apparently senseless happening by providing a causal and moral explanation (Mayer 1970:50). One interviewee told me:

> Some people readily suspect sorcery because for many years they have been faithful to their spouse. But suddenly they got sick. It *must* be something like sorcery!

Across different cultures, the "why him/why her" question is usually explained in personal terms, based on the assumption that certain people intervene in the fortunes of others.[5] "There is always somebody responsible" (Berglund 1989:109). Various comments in my interviews support the argument that some personal agency must be responsible for misfortune and ill-health:

> In our tradition we believe that a human being does not die naturally but is killed! It does not matter how old the person is, in our tradition a human being is killed by someone. It is said that no one just dies; an individual is murdered by a sorcerer!

There is another way of looking at such views. In Zimbabwe, as in many other cultures, identifying the culprit offers some hope for changing the fate of the victim. It thus becomes possible to deal with misfortune and suffering. This is important for understanding sorcery beliefs in relation to AIDS. Western medicine cannot provide a cure for HIV/AIDS, thus death becomes inevitable.

The unavailability and unaffordability of ARV drugs, as well as the decaying public healthcare system, only further such perceptions. Sorcery offers a way to cope with these depressing healthcare conditions, promising a possible cure by identifying the sorcerer and counteracting the evil force.[6] When HIV/AIDS is interpreted within the sorcery paradigm, a terminal condition is transformed in a treatable one. This argument also applies to conspiracy theories; identifying the conspirator makes it possible to stop the suffering of AIDS.

Across cultures, people recognize that illness and death can result from natural causes (for instance, old age) even though some individuals may still interpret the death of an elder to be the result of sorcery (Malinowski 1969:187). People understand some illnesses and their causes in biomedical terms, grouping them together into two broad categories.[7] The first contains diseases regarded as normal or natural, usually minor ailments such as the common cold. In Zimbabwe, as elsewhere, even HIV/AIDS is at times seen as a natural disease caused by an invisible biological agent within the bloodstream and bones of the body.[8] The earlier stages of AIDS are more readily interpreted in terms of a natural disease because their symptoms come and go, and medical treatment appears to be successful.

Full-blown AIDS, however, appears unnatural because the able-bodied, or the young and strong, suffer a terminal disease (Ashforth 2002:131; Drew et al. 1996:81). AIDS symptoms appear abnormal because they persist over a long time, do not positively respond to treatment, and recur. In many societies this pattern raises suspicions that some unnatural agent is responsible—something suspicious is happening (e.g., Kluckhohn 1944:82). It has been said that such a slow, wasting disease is a clear sign of a sorcerer at work (Evans-Pritchard 1976b:14; Green 1999:34). We should not be surprised that HIV/AIDS, which exhibits such dismal patterns of disease progression, is interpreted in Zimbabwe and elsewhere in terms of sorcery.

Scholars argue that the increasing incidence of AIDS results in a proliferation of sorcery suspicions (Anderson 2002:432). Although I did not observe a proliferation of sorcery accusations in Zimbabwe between 1991 and 2003, respondents frequently mentioned sorcery to explain AIDS. One interviewee said:

> AIDS is really a satanic disease because no one dies of it without suspicions being raised that they were bewitched by someone.

Traditional diviners, as well as prophets of some indigenous churches, are called upon to identify the culprit. Such a search triggers animosities. This is why the interviewee called AIDS a "satanic" disease. People stop trusting each other, begin suspecting that someone is out to harm them, and want to identify this evil person. Anthropologists have observed that sorcery is often built on terror, producing fear and stress rather than satisfaction, and may even disturb amicable social relations (de Blécourt 1999:208–209; Schoepf 1991:756). Support for such an argument comes from my interviews:

> The truth is that many people end up hating each other and suspect that some are plotting something evil. But to say the truth, nothing

is plotted; it is just our heart that is suspicious. AIDS has caused so many suspicions that divide the community!

Interpreting HIV/AIDS as an unnatural disease caused by sorcery disrupts society in several ways. Those suffering full-blown AIDS victimize others in the community as they desperately search for cause and cure. Clinging to the sorcery paradigm gives temporary hope to AIDS sufferers that there may be a reversal of their suffering, but at the same time it does violence to those accused of being the sorcerers. This is not happening only in Zimbabwe.

It does appear that sorcery beliefs about HIV/AIDS are causing friction within communities. However, since Malinowski (1926:94) described the value of sorcery in the culture of the Trobriand islanders, anthropologists have noted the positive side of some sorcery beliefs and practices across cultures. Their observations are relevant to the interpretation of the AIDS epidemic within the sorcery paradigm.

Scholars frequently cite as a function of sorcery beliefs the maintenance of social cohesion and enforcing of social norms and values.[9] This function becomes evident when we look at the selection of those accused. Across cultures, a fundamental distinction of sorcerers into insiders and outsiders occurs (Douglas 1970:xxvi–xxvii). When the sorcerer is an outsider, sorcery beliefs reaffirm group boundaries and solidarity by casting blame for misfortune outside.[10] In Zimbabwe this applies more to conspiracy theories than to sorcery beliefs. The outsider-conspirator is generally seen as a powerful stranger. Zimbabwean and regional politicians—aware that fear of a threat from outside can rally support among the electorate, and to unify a divided nation—frequently referred to AIDS conspiracies.

In contrast, the insider-sorcerer is portrayed as a debased individual, whose behavior is characterized by profound immorality, selfishness, and greed.[11] The accused are those who are weak and who have few supporters. They are less likely to fight back when they are accused of sorcery arising from their immorality.[12] Not surprisingly, most people with whom I spoke expressed their conviction that women, elders, and members of minority groups are the most likely to engage in sorcery—including sorcery that gives meaning to the AIDS epidemic.

Yet, sometimes the opposite seems to be the case, and suspicion is directed toward older, affluent men, some of whom hold important positions in society (Kluckhohn 1944:6, 111). In Zimbabwe, for example, the *undofa* belief is associated with the successful. The affluent and powerful who are deemed sorcerers are seen as having enriched themselves with the help of the *undofa*-familiar. Such accusations are lodged against individuals who refuse to share their wealth with others. Assigning them this negative attribute is a strong appeal to them to show concern for other members of the social group. In these situations the use of the term *sorcerer* may be entirely metaphorical.

The question whether an accusation is meant literally or metaphorically is crucial to understanding the dynamics of attributing blame for misfortune. Sorcery is, across cultures, a widespread source of metaphors for talking about antisocial and immoral behavior (Ellen 1993:20–21). This became apparent during my discussions with Zimbabweans. The following are typical examples:

> Of course there are sorcerers, I know them, but I do not believe that a sorcerer is able to cause AIDS. I do not believe this except when the sorcerer, who is a human being like us, can infect you with HIV through sexual intercourse.

> The disease-of-these-days[13] exists. It is a reality. The sorcerers just take advantage of its existence. The sorcerer can also cause you to have AIDS! The sorcerer can take a razor, cut a person who is HIV-positive, and then come to you during the night and cut you with the same razor.

These interviewees speak of knowingly and deliberately infecting others with HIV. My data contain many references to evil-minded individuals who know that they are HIV-positive but still continue to have sexual intercourse with their marital and extramarital partners. These individuals are (metaphorically) being called sorcerers! Naming as sorcerers those who flout the community's values functions as a social control and is a way of teaching what is acceptable behavior and what is not.

Anthropologists have also observed that, across cultures, sorcery suspicions—far beyond enforcing social norms and strengthening social cohesion—address tense relationships and disputes between individuals.[14] Sorcery accusations arise out of interpersonal conflict, not only out of deviance from definable community norms. Particularly in small, face-to-face communities, where it is difficult to disperse ill feeling that results from ordinary social life, sorcery suspicions occur. Individuals and groups turn to sorcery beliefs when other means of relieving tensions are either exhausted or not applicable. As such, sorcery responses are "social-strain-gauges" [a phrase coined by Marwick] that enable individuals to address social tension that otherwise could not be as easily addressed (Marwick 1963:13). They allow for the release of aggressive impulses without serious threat to the social fabric.

Statements about sorcery in Nkulumane clearly support an interpretation of such beliefs and practices in terms of social strains that are not easily addressed otherwise. People argued that in times of misfortune they are especially suspicious of those with whom they have a strained relationship because cultural expectations of showing respect make it difficult to solve the relationship problem easily. The following is an example of this dynamic:

> We buried one of my nephews last December. He told me that he
> visited his father and removed his shoes in the field to do some work
> for him. Afterward, when he wore the shoes, he felt a sudden pain
> in his feet. He suspected something sinister and started blaming his
> father for plotting to harm him. It is so common that someone who
> has AIDS blames others for it. My nephew thought that his own father
> was killing him because of problems between them.

This case is unusual in that the son accused his own father of having used sorcery against him. In the patrilineal Ndebele society, father and son belong to the same kin group, and such accusations are generally expressed across different lines of kinship. Targeting members of one's own lineage would anger the family's ancestors, who would likely withdraw their protection from the sorcerer (Ngubane 1976:330). But this example represents a case of sorcery that functions as a social-strain-gauge. The son's behavior toward the father is heavily determined by cultural patterns of showing respect. The son would have had difficulty expressing problems with his father. His illness, which was AIDS-related, allowed him to use the sorcery paradigm to speak about the troubled relationship with his parent. He traced his illness to an "accident," a sorcery attack by his father.

My discussions with Zimbabweans show that it is more common that suspicions target individuals from other kin groups, such as non-lineage members of the household, or in-laws. The following exemplifies the tendency to raise sorcery accusations when relationships are strained between individuals who are not kin:

> Especially when the husband gets sick, his mother will say that the son's wife caused the disease. Likewise, when the wife is sick, her family will claim that the husband is responsible for the disease of their daughter. There are a lot of mutual accusations.

The relationships between a spouse and the parents-in-law are strongly shaped by notions of respect. Among some Zimbabwean ethnic groups the son-in-law does not eat in the presence of his mother-in-law, rarely speaks unless asked, and covers his shoulders in her presence. It is difficult for him to express any difficulties he has with her. Similar patterns apply also to the relationships of a woman with her mother-in-law. Sorcery accusations between them provide an outlet for addressing difficult relationships that are not easily addressed otherwise. We can see these dynamics at work in other relationships. People may designate any difficult person as the responsible aggressor when misfortune occurs. The sorcery paradigm is a way of framing such suspicions.

Stress caused by challenging economic, political, and other conditions leads to social tension. Competition for a highly valued goal connected with such fields of aspiration as leadership, property, jobs, or love generates tension leading to sorcery suspicions.[15] Cross-culturally, individuals perceive emotions and attitudes of envy, jealousy, and greed to be the basic motivation for engaging in sorcery.[16] My interview data provide ample evidence that jealousy and greed are seen as the most likely motivations underlying sorcery. One informant said:

> Sorcery is jealousy. For instance, I want to get rid of you and remain behind alone, enjoying the pleasures of life without sharing them with you.

A core characteristic of sorcery is to gain something from others through hurting or even killing them. The driving forces behind such behavior are jealousy and greed, emotions that affect people more strongly during times of hardship and social unrest. When I did fieldwork in Zimbabwe, high unemployment, a galloping inflation, and severe continuing shortages of even the most basic commodities made life difficult.[17] The frightening reality resulted in competition over resources and in envy among individuals, providing a fertile ground for sorcery arguments, including some involving HIV/AIDS beliefs. Nkulumane residents said that:

> It happens frequently that families deny that their relatives are dying of AIDS. Instead they argue that someone must be jealous because they have been promoted in their jobs.

> My mother-in-law said, "Yes, my son was sick, but there is a reason for his sickness!" She thought that someone in his work did not like him, wanted to get his job, and bewitched him. In his case it was obvious that he was dying of AIDS, but she did not want to believe it.

These quotes indicate patterns for the diagnosis of misfortune when the suffering individuals would have attracted envy. Conversely, in identifying the sorcerer people tend to look for individuals who would benefit from sorcery (Farmer 1992:70, 87).

Early scholarship on sorcery recognized that sorcery has strong economic implications (Kluckhohn 1944). Over time, scholars have supported this finding, pointing out that sorcery may balance socioeconomic inequality through accumulative and leveling tendencies (Geschiere 1997:208).

Sorcery may provide indispensable support for the dominant to accumulate greater wealth and influence. Cross-culturally, and throughout history, sorcery accusations were used as a means to defend, protect, and reinforce social inequality by accusing the subordinate of evil intent, thus neutralizing a potential threat to the powerful and ensuring compliance and conformity.[18] My observations in Zimbabwe did not unearth AIDS beliefs that could be interpreted in this line of thought. This tendency appeared more akin to some conspiracy theories that were promoted by local politicians. As mentioned earlier, people argued that governing politicians are implicated in the unabated spread of the AIDS epidemic. Accused politicians defused such accusations by pointing at outside culprits, thus cementing their political power by identifying a common enemy.

All over the world, sorcery can be seen as a leveling influence, a weapon used by the weak to make the powerful fulfill their obligation to the powerless of society.[19] Fear of being accused of sorcery promotes charitable behavior of the powerful toward the subordinated. My data strongly support this argument. For instance, a participant in a focus group discussion made the following statement echoing similar sentiments:

> The old women, who see that we are successful in life and even own cars, intrigue against us by saying that we young professionals use sorcery, and even cause AIDS, in order to become successful and rich.

The "old women" who depend on their younger relatives and offspring for support may indeed accuse them of accumulating wealth through sorcery practices and inflicting harm on others—even a terminal disease like HIV/AIDS. Presumably the women intend their accusation to force a sharing of the wealth. In Plumtree, such accusations did trigger fear in the more affluent. I met an elderly man who, by local standards, was economically successful. He had managed to extend his house, acquire cattle for his small farm plot, keep goats and chickens, and buy a pickup truck. One of his daughters was living in Switzerland and another one in

Britain. By local standards, he fared extremely well. Neighbors and relatives often approached him for financial help, which he refused. The rumor spread that he was a sorcerer who had accumulated his wealth with the help of an *undofa*. Anthropologists have observed similar dynamics across diverse cultures;[20] the accumulation of wealth is a central characteristic in sorcery beliefs across diverse cultures (Favret-Saada 1989:42–43).

Anthropologists during the last decades argued that sorcery is a symbolic expression of the problem of evil in a context of rapid social, political, and economic change (e.g., Comaroff and Comaroff 1993, 1998). They saw sorcery as persisting in modernity, global capitalism, and accelerating changes. People during change frequently return to traditional beliefs and behaviors to reassert a measure of control. While these studies do not part with their predecessors' argument that sorcery is a response to some sort of stress,[21] they insist that sorcery operates as part and parcel of modernity itself. Such theoretical insights have been applied to sorcery suspicions as they arose in the AIDS epidemic (e.g., Devisch 2001:102).

Despite the interpretive value of such arguments, these studies do not focus on the genealogy of sorcery in specific communities, instead generalizing a vast body of evidence, while losing sight of other social processes that contribute to the evolution of sorcery beliefs besides the global economy (Behringer 2004:29; Rutherford 1999:91–92, 97). Arguments that situate sorcery beliefs within modernity are nevertheless important for an *etic* analysis of sorcery beliefs. However, my discussions with Zimbabweans show that people's *emic* interpretations of sorcery beliefs do not relate sorcery to wider macroeconomic issues.

In day-to-day life, sorcery deals with the individuals and issues affecting them directly, such as the competition for scarce jobs and jealousy within the workplace. Though wider economic forces create the conditions that cause personal strain for individuals, these macroeconomic forces are, at least in my data, not believed to be related to sorcery. My data indicate that global forces beyond the local are more explicitly addressed in conspiracy theories. Traditional sorcery beliefs, however, are expressed when the life of an individual is at stake.

We now look more closely at sorcery beliefs that people invoke as an explanation for the suffering of HIV/AIDS. Some studies indicate that AIDS deaths are frequently blamed on sorcery while other studies across sub-Saharan Africa report far fewer incidences.[22] There may be varying reasons for this discrepancy, including their selection of methods (see Chapter 1). Still, as differences have been reported, we need to examine the frequency of placing blame for AIDS in Zimbabwe.

During my discussions with Zimbabweans, explicit denials of the importance of sorcery in the causation of AIDS occasionally emerged. Some residents in Nkulumane asserted that AIDS has nothing to do with sorcery. For instance, one interviewee flatly said:

A sorcerer is not able to give me AIDS. AIDS is different from sorcery.

People observed that the pattern of HIV-infection differs from the way individuals are affected by ailments caused by sorcery. The most commonly observed difference is that AIDS spreads rapidly from one person to another while sorcery targets only intended victims. People realized that a certain individual falls ill and dies, and then is followed by the spouse. People do know of certain sorcery practices that affect members of the same extended family, who may die one after another.

An example of such sorcery is the raising of avenging spirits, the so-called *ngozi* (Schoormann 2005: 466–78). This type of traditional sorcery largely affects members of a single lineage; among the patrilineal ethnic groups in Zimbabwe the wife belongs to a different lineage and would not be affected by this type of sorcery. Another example is *ulunyoka*, a sorcery practice that is not believed to attack both spouses. Chapter 5 elaborates on this practice.

An exception from the pattern that sorcery does not affect spouses is the belief that HIV is transmitted through an *undofa* to one of the spouses, and then from that spouse to the other spouse. (Chapter 4 describes the *undofa*.) However, overall it is rather unusual for sorcery practices to affect individuals of different lineages and to spread quickly from one person to another. AIDS, in contrast, usually affects both husband and wife, and through them, others.

Furthermore, though some traditional sorcery maladies have a relation to illicit sex, people observed that HIV/AIDS is primarily a sexually transmitted disease while sorcery-induced ailments are not perceived as STDs alone. Those rumored to be promiscuous are thought to be the first ones dying of AIDS. Frequently residents made these statements during interviews:

> The death of this young man has nothing to do with sorcery. He was just very fast. This is what killed him.

> Individuals with AIDS are just careless with their bodies. This is the problem and not sorcery.

Being "fast" and "careless" are euphemisms for being promiscuous. A similar idea was expressed by saying that people who "move around a lot" are the ones who acquire HIV. AIDS was first associated with movement, mobility, and travel, and later became associated with promiscuity. *Fast* and *careless* seem to be common expressions in southern and eastern African languages as people argue that HIV/AIDS spreads rapidly because so many are promiscuous.[23]

The recent appearance and wide distribution of the AIDS epidemic further discredits an interpretation that AIDS-related ailments are due to sorcery:

> Sorcery has always been around, but it has never been as widespread as AIDS. AIDS is much more widespread. AIDS is just a disease.

While some scholars indicate that the high incidence of AIDS results in high incidence of sorcery suspicions (Ashforth 2002), some of my informants argue the very fact that AIDS is so widespread actually discredits its interpretation in terms of sorcery; for them, the reference to sorcery makes sense only for a few individual cases. They see no reasons for assuming that sorcery is more widespread now than in the past. Therefore, HIV/AIDS is something else, most probably just a disease, though a "new" disease.

Various traditional healers corroborated this view. They argued during interviews that the ancestors fail to tell them how to cure someone with this disease because the ancestors had never encountered the disease. The ancestors can only compare the symptoms of the new disease with those of old diseases and recommend appropriate medicinals and dosages to treat the symptoms. The ancestors do not know how to cure AIDS completely. Informants who observed that traditional medicine is unable to completely cure AIDS-related symptoms conclude that explaining the condition through reference to sorcery is doubtful:

> Despite suspecting sorcery and pointing fingers at particular individuals, the sick person sometimes still dies. In the end, it was just a disease and not sorcery. But some family members will still continue explaining AIDS in terms of sorcery.

People who follow this line of argument generally conclude that HIV/AIDS is transmitted by a virus. We must keep in mind, however, that such views are usually *outsiders'* perspectives. As argued earlier, people shift their explanatory strategies according to the situation. Those directly affected by the epidemic may remain suspicious that sorcery is at work despite evidence to the contrary.

During interviews, some Zimbabweans did refer to sorcery when explaining HIV/AIDS. This association of HIV with sorcery seems to be more common among people who are either infected with HIV or have an AIDS sufferer in the family. Though they may honestly believe such explanations, other residents explain the higher incidence of sorcery attribution with HIV/AIDS through its association with illicit sexual behavior:

> Sick individuals were hiding the fact that they have this disease because of shame. This is because the disease is acquired through sex. In other words, the sick person is thought to be a prostitute, someone who does not have a proper moral conduct. Therefore, to speak about AIDS is an insult to the sick person. When people see that their relative is sick, they strongly suspect the person of poor moral conduct. They hide the person away, because it is embarrassing for them. Or, they deny that the sickness is AIDS, saying that the patient simply has persistent headache, chest problems, or something else.

As the association of AIDS with culturally inappropriate sexual behavior is so strong, the attribution of blame to the AIDS sufferer is common. In southern Zimbabwe the disease is popularly called *umkuhlane wesiwule* (whoring disease). Prostitutes and those having sexual intercourse with them are assumed to be infected with HIV. More generally, HIV/AIDS is called *ingculaza*. Some explained that this term has two meanings: first, it connotes that AIDS is the disease that makes people dirty (derived from the verb *ukungcola*, "to be dirty") and second, that AIDS, like the Spanish influenza *iyachola*, "grinds" and "destroys" the whole nation.[24]

Because of these negative meanings for HIV/AIDS, many avoid explicit mention of it, saying instead that someone has *umkhuhlane lo* ("this disease") or "TB-II." In the first years of the epidemic, AIDS sufferers were often hidden away and left to die unattended because their families were shamed. When others asked about the sick individual, minor ailments were cited as the cause of the illness.

As the AIDS epidemic has come to affect nearly every household directly or indirectly, the issue of shame and secrecy has decreased to some extent. Nevertheless, the negative connotations attached to the disease still make it difficult to speak openly about it, particularly when a family member develops full-blown AIDS. Subsequently the illness may be blamed on sorcery:

> Many people have AIDS, but when *my* child[25] has the disease, then I say the child is bewitched, although I see with my own eyes that the suffering is due to AIDS. Only a few admit that it is due to AIDS. It is easier to admit AIDS with other people. When a neighbor's child is affected, then people blame it on AIDS.

A reference to sorcery implicitly locates the blame outside the individual. An important function of sorcery arguments is to exonerate persons of guilt from having done something wrong. The condition is blamed on others (Krige 1970:250; Kluckhohn 1944:99). For this reason those affected by AIDS, or their relatives, are more inclined to invoke sorcery as the precipitating cause. The socially stigmatized disease is replaced by a socially acceptable one.[26] This may be expressed by anyone within the social group of the suffering individuals or by the individuals themselves.

Local writers picked up this theme. Among them was Nzenza-Shand, who wrote about the suffering and death of a young man:

> Patrick's parents could not believe that their mission-educated boy could have been sleeping with prostitutes. They felt that if this *hedzi*[27] existed, it should affect other people—surely not their handsome boy. They started to believe that their son had an evil spell cast on him by someone in the village or someone jealous of his success. (Nzenza-Shand 1997:11–12)

The shameful association of HIV/AIDS with illicit sex motivated Patrick's parents to search for alternative explanations. While the stigma of illicit sex may bring sorcery beliefs forward in many instances, in others people seem to be genuinely convinced that sorcery is responsible for an individual's suffering.

I formed the impression from my interviews that people often believed sorcery accusations to be true. Naturally, they resolved to use the appropriate channels for addressing sorcery suspicions. First, they contacted a diviner to identify the culprit and the medicines for both treatment and protection. An informant related the following story to me that succinctly summarizes such sentiments within a family:

> The brother of my husband, who was successful in life and lived somewhere else, had a relationship with another woman. It was one of those women who need to be advised or even brought to court. So, he visited this lady from time to time but afterward always went back to his wife. He "tasted the sweet honey" here and there. Then he became sick. He started coughing but his health improved again. When he finally died suspicions of sorcery were raised about the cause of his death. After he died, his wife, although she knew of his immoral behavior, said that she herself feels weak at times and suspects the mother-in-law to have bewitched her.

Although the informant respectfully says that this married man had a relationship with a woman, I suspected that the person actually meant that the man was having sexual relations with prostitutes. The expressions that this woman "needs to be advised" or "brought to court" points at her loose lifestyle; the terms are euphemisms for prostitution, which is prohibited in Zimbabwe. The fact that the married man was successful in life shows that he was able to pay for sex. And the expression that he "tasted the sweet honey," the pleasure of the sexual encounter, "here and there" can be interpreted as having more than one sexual partner. It was evident that he acquired HIV through extramarital sexual behavior that finally developed into full-blown AIDS.

Two lines of sorcery suspicions were actually expressed. First, following the man's death, his family raised suspicions targeting his wife. In many cases wives are the first to be accused. The second line of suspicions began when the wife fell ill and claimed her mother-in-law had bewitched her. Close individuals outside one's own lineage are usually the first suspects. Other such examples in the study revealed that many residents firmly believed in the possibility that acts of sorcery are responsible for HIV/AIDS.

Zimbabweans, as with people elsewhere, did not agree on the interpretation of AIDS as the result of sorcerers' practices. Disagreement applied to general patterns of sorcery already discussed. When people talked about specific sorcery beliefs and practices in interviews, it became clear that research must inquire into such specifics and their emic interpretations. The next two chapters discuss the three methods of aggression commonly identified by interviewees.

Notes

1. This argument has been brought forward by scholars in various disciplines, including Ashforth 2005:xiii; Behringer 2004:17; Kluckhohn 1944:122; and Middleton and Winter 1963:1.
2. A plethora of literature supports this argument, e.g., Blyth-Whiting 1950:33; Bowden 1987:183; Darling 1999:738; Foster 1976:773; Good 1987:93; Hoebel 1952:388; Joralemon and Douglas 1993:196; Kleivan 1984:618; Rodman 1979:5; and Scaletta 1985:232.

3. This point was made by various anthropologists, for example, Beidelman 1970:351; Kapferer 1997:10; Larner 1981:7; MacFarlane 1970:3; Marwick 1970; Stephen 1987a:2–7; and Whitehead 2002:205.

4. Lemert 1997:20 and Middleton and Winter 1963:2 are critical of the cross-cultural applicability of this distinction. In contrast, some sort of distinction has been documented by, e.g., Berglund 1976:266–67; Darling 1999:735; Hammond-Tooke 1993:169–71; Hoebel 1952:388; Kluckhohn 1944:22–45; Leiban 1967:20, 65; and Saler 1964:320–22. Some scholars supporting some sort of distinction point out that the conceptual distinction is not reflected in a linguistic distinction, e.g., Berglund 1976:266–67 and Crawford 1967:141.

5. For a more thorough discussion on this point, see Berglund 1976:270; Bond and Ciekawy 2001:6; Douglas 1966:98; Gluckman 1970:326–27; and Kluckhohn 1944:87.

6. This function of sorcery has been pointed out, e.g., by Bourdillon 1993:110; Crawford 1967:69; and Kluckhohn 1944:107.

7. See, e.g., Ashforth 2005:45; Chavunduka 1986:32; Murray and Alvarez 1973:12; and Ngubane 1976:322.

8. This is a common perception in southern Africa as documented, e.g., by Green 1999:39; Le Beau 2002:98; and Wolf 1996a:153. People with whom I talked sometimes called a disease agent *isibungu*, referring to a small insect, maggot, worm, or beetle. More appropriately, people called it *igciwane*, the extremely small, invisible living being in the body. At times they attached "HIV," *igciwane leHIV*, to clearly express which disease agent they were talking about.

9. This view has been widely argued, e.g., by Appel 1977:76; Beidelman 1963:96–97; Brain 1975:186; Chowning 1987:149, 177; Douglas 1970:xxvi–xxvii; Epstein 1974:18; Evans-Pritchard 1976b:50; Forge 1970:273; Kilpatrick 1997:10; Kluckhohn 1944:110–13; Lamphere 1971:107; Leiban 1967:125, 149; Lemert 1997:19; Lindenbaum 1981:123; Madsen and Madsen 1989:236; Marwick 1963:20; 1965:245; Sidky 1997:256; Spindler 1989:63; Stephen 1987a:10; and Walker 1989:7.

10. For more on the outsider-sorcerer see, e.g., Forge 1970:258; Gonzales 1989:285–86; Marwick 1970:280–81; Patterson 1974/75:149–59; and Reay 1987a:113–14.

11. For more on the insider-sorcerer see, e.g., Auslander 1993:178; Bond 2001:143–55; Lemert 1997:45; Mayer 1970:60–61; Pollock 1996:331; and Taussig 1980:117.

12. There is a lot written about factors determining the selection of a suspected sorcerer, e.g., Blyth-Whiting 1950:64–66; Carneiro 1977:227; Estes 1985:246; Lemert 1997:47, 102; Mary Aquina 1968:48; Meursing 1997:144; Reay 1987b:113; Sidky 1997:258; and Stewart and Strathern 2004:ix.

13. This term is another euphemism for AIDS.

14. A rich and variegated body of literature exists on this function of sorcery beliefs, for instance, Ashforth 2005:71; Beidelman 1970:354; Brain 1970:162; Chavunduka 1982:6; Golomb 1985:182; Hunter-Wilson 1970:263; Leiban 1967:5; Lemert 1997:46; LeVine 1982:279; Marwick 1967:125; Mavhungu 2002:68; Mayer 1970:46; Nadel 1970:278; 1978:28; Obeyesekere 1975:19; Pollock 1996:330; Stephen 1987a:6; Stewart and Strathern 2004:9; Turner 1964:324, 1968:46–47; and Westerlund 1989:171.

15. The argument that sorcery suspicions are triggered by societal problems leading to competition is brought forward, e.g., by Anderson 2002:245–46; Beattie 1963:49–50; Bourdillon 1993:118; Darling 1999:735; Dillon-Malone 1988; Le Beau 2002:94–98; Madsen and Madsen 1989:236; Marwick 1952:127–30, 1963:21; Middleton and Winter 1963:20–21; Mitchell 1960:194; Silverblatt 1987:186–96; Steadman 1985:121–22; and Walker 1989:3–4.

16. Envy and jealousy as emotions fostering sorcery suspicions are mentioned in a wide range of literature, e.g., Ashforth 2000:50–51; Balikci 1984:425; Behringer 2004:244; Berglund 1976:272, 315, 287; de Blécourt 1999:206; Gluckman 1965:235–36; Kaetzler 2001:79–94; Menegoni 1996:392; Ncube 2003; Niehaus 2001:128; Pelton 1992:23; Reynolds 1990:327; Saler 1964:312; Segar 1997a, 1997b:209; Selby 1974:108; and Turner 1968:47, 1981:146. Some years ago a traditional healer in Salzburg, Austria, explained to me that envy can be a powerful means to inflict illness on others. She explained multiple sclerosis, for instance, as being caused because someone close to the ill individual is envious of him or her.

17. Farmer made the observation that sorcery is triggered in societies that experience situations of scarcity resulting in high competition (1992:204–206).

18. The accumulative tendency of sorcery is mentioned, e.g., by Bailey 1994:3; Harris 1975:240; Niehaus 2001:10, 112; Sidky 1997:260–65; and Stewart and Strathern 2004:15.

19. The leveling tendency of sorcery is discussed, e.g., in Darling 1999:743; Douglas 1980:49; Evans-Pritchard 1976b:54-55; Kluckhohn 1944:228–29; Loeb 1929:83; Sweet 2003:187; and Yamba 1997:218. Such literature follows the line of thought that the subordinated use means of resistance against their oppressors. See Scott 1985:169.

20. See, e.g., Behringer 2004:28; Farmer 1992:11; Geschiere 1998; Meyer 1995; Offiong 1991; and van der Drift 1992.

21. This has been argued by scholars in various academic traditions, e.g., by Behringer 2004:212; Dillon-Malone 1988:1162; Evans-Pritchard 1929:636; Malinowski 1963:261, 1969:197–98; Parrinder 1963:205; and Scholz-Williams 1995:3

22. For example, these studies found widespread evidence of such beliefs: Kasule et al. 1997:79; Ndubani 1998:2; and Sankara 1995. The following, in contrast, encountered less evidence: Bernstein and van Rooyen 1994:377; Caprara et al. 1993:1231; Forster 1998:539–42; and Setel 1999:219.

23. Support for this argument comes, e.g., from Mogensen 1997:437; Setel 1999:212; and Yamba 1997:206.

24. The interpretations given are from township residents. However, the term is explained differently in the literature. *Ingcolaze,* the Zulu variant of the Ndebele *ingculaza,* is used in the context of the local concept of taboo, *inhlonipho* (Huyssteyn 2002:220–21). Respect, honor, and reverence are shown through the use of substitute terms. An offensive term is replaced by an inoffensive expression. *Inhlonipho* thus led to the coining of the Zulu term *ingcolaze* for HIV/AIDS, to avoid speaking directly of AIDS. The new term is a compound of the word for a poison used to kill the chief of a Zulu king, *umgcalaza,* and the term for sexual transmitted diseases, *ugcunsula.*

25. In this and the following quote, "child" does not refer to a minor; it refers to an adult who is a "child" in relation to an elder in the family. It indicates the positioning of the addressee within a structure of authority and respect in relation to the speaker.

26. This seems to be a common pattern cross-culturally. See, e.g., McMillen 2004:898–99; Munk 1997:11; Niehaus and Jonssen 2005:180–81; Schoormann 2005:359; and Yamba 1997:217.

27. Literal transcription of AIDS into the Shona language.

CHAPTER 4

A Sorcerer's Servant-Being

In the beginning of my research, respondents told me that sorcerers use *ondofa*, servant-beings that are typical of familiars recognized in reports of sorcery from many cultures.[1] *Ondofa* carry out the sorcerers' orders, helping to accumulate wealth and to punish enemies. Though experienced sorcerers are the most likely to use these beings, anyone can obtain them and turn into a sorcerer. Some Zimbabweans expressed firm belief in *ondofa*. A middle-aged woman said:

> The *ondofa* are a reality. Even on TV we are told that the *ondofa* are alive.

The influence of the media is apparent in this quote; mass media have influenced the spread of modern sorcery globally (Behringer 2004:237). The media are reinforcing the sorcery beliefs of many residents in the township where I worked. Yet, my observations indicate that the media are even more influential on the development of conspiracy beliefs.

Although a few people denied the existence of the *ondofa*, they still debated their actual visibility. People said that these creatures are elusive; they are seen mainly at night or at twilight. Several informants said they have glimpsed one or more *ondofa*, usually only for a short time because the familiars ran away and hid. I remember one young man saying that he saw one several times in the early hours of the day when fog blurred visibility. A middle-aged woman related how she had seen one resting on a Durawall (precast cement panels commonly used to fence a yard). Seeing her, the *undofa* immediately jumped down and scurried into hiding. Generally people agreed that *ondofa* are less active in daylight or under streetlights.

In interviews I was told that the *ondofa* are "grown" from "roots" treated in a particular way:

> A friend of mine obtained a bottle with something in it that looked like a small piece of wood, but he couldn't clearly see what it was. People tell us that these are "roots." My friend was told to lay the bottle on a cupboard; the piece would then start germinating and finally grow into a human being. My friend was very surprised to see that this actually happened and that, after some time, a human-like creature was in the bottle.

In other parts of the region, people described sorcery methods that required the use of substances such as animal fats, blood, and other ingredients (sometimes a human spirit) to create an *undofa*. This echoes methods to obtain other locally known familiars, such as the *umkhoba*, which is produced by capturing the soul of a deceased person, or by resuscitating a dead individual, or even by taming an offspring of a sorcerer and a baboon. The belief the creature can be "produced" with the help of some human spirit, situates these familiars within comparable zombie phenomena in other regions.[2] However, the main ingredient for an *undofa* is a "root," which somehow mysteriously develops into the creature. *Root* is commonly understood in southern Africa to be another term for medicinals and has the same ambiguous meaning as *umuthi,* which was described earlier.

The *ondofa* and related beings have a relatively uniform appearance, with similar characteristics and behaviors, throughout southern Africa.[3] They are generally thought to be short, hairy, male creatures that have some resemblance to baboons that walk on two legs, but at times I was told some of them are female, capable of producing offspring. While the male *undofa* has an extraordinarily large member, the female has extremely large breasts. Artist Sheunesu Shumba made a carving of a typical male *undofa*, omitting the exaggerated genitalia out of decency, as he told me (right).

The great value of *ondofa* is that they accumulate wealth for their owners (Crawford 1967:119; Kaetzler 2001:88–89), a central characteristic of sorcery cross-culturally, as argued earlier. To enrich their owners, *ondofa* move around the township and beyond to steal money and possessions. Their presence means trouble in a neighborhood when residents realize an *undofa* is around. Householders hear strange, persistent noises during the night, find belongings to be missing, and are even struck in the dark.

Ondofa are thought to be clever. They can act as good luck charms, luring customers to shops and thus creating wealth for the shopkeepers. Descriptions vary somewhat. At times, as respondents described it, *ondofa* simply work for their owners, for

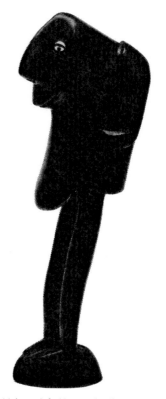

Male *undofa*. (Carving by Sheunesu Shumba. Photo by Heinz Helf.)

example with familiars such as snakes or baboons. Any creature could potentially become a sorcerer's familiar, through magic, to serve the owner's purposes. The strong connections people perceive between these creatures and the accumulation of wealth is associated with the rapid economic progress of the *ondofa's* owners. Nowadays the wealthy people in the townships tend to be those who work in South Africa or Botswana. People explain that Zimbabwean migrant laborers obtained the "root" to produce an *undofa* in South Africa (see also Anderson 2002:430):

> Well, I was told that it is a small thing which you can get in South Africa. It is usually kept at home, especially by those who go often to South Africa. The migrant laborers who go to South Africa have them.

Many of these migrant laborers support their families with their earnings. Especially at Christmas, many return home ostentatiously displaying their newly gained wealth. Migrant laborers not only return with their new riches, but also with *ondofa*. People agree that the workers must have accumulated their wealth through illegitimate means. Such suspicions may function as an appeal to share, echoing what was said in Chapter 3 about the leveling tendency of some sorcery suspicions. Sharing wealth dispels accusations that the successful individual is a greedy and selfish sorcerer.

Accumulating wealth with the help of a familiar has its risks. Although the creature serves humans, it is understood to have its own will. It can act independently. It may even turn against its owner, if the owner fails to care for it properly. In exchange for the familiar's labor, the *undofa* expects food and shelter. If owners fail to reciprocate, familiars might beat them or even chase them away. This indicates that the *undofa* belongs to a particular type of familiars.

While familiars of one type are sent by the sorcerer to particular persons and strictly follow the sorcerer's wishes, familiars of another type, including the *undofa*, exhibit a certain autonomy. Though at times they act as instruments of their owner's malevolent desires and ambitions, at other times they override their owner's wishes (Turner 1968:14). The sorcerer accepts this risk because of a desire to accumulate wealth by any means without scruples. The sorcerer's greed goes so far that it endangers the life of others:

> The creature stays in the home and destroys your family. Now you see the problem of getting rich—it destroys your family. For you to get rich, others have to suffer. So it is better to remain poor.

> The creature will look for money for you. I as a woman need money. We women want a lot of things! We say that our children are dying, killed by money. Money is the root of all evil.

These creatures can make their owners rich, but they are a dangerous burden that may not be worth the wealth they bring. The *ondofa* harm others and can even destroy the owner's family. The word *kill* was used in the second interview in the metaphorical sense of hurting others; it is generally said that someone is "killing" someone else when a possession, or an opportunity to gain something, is taken away from that person by someone else.

Another common metaphorical expression for inflicting harm is to *eat* someone. Cross-culturally, such expressions do not refer to cannibalism as such but are often general references to harming others (Murray and Alvarez 1973:40). The expressions reflect the belief that one person's gain is another's loss; others have to suffer because of the greed of one person. At times this expression is taken literally; wealth is not only obtained by taking it from someone else but even by literally sacrificing someone. This is evidenced in other parts of the world,[4] but it was also recorded by Nzenza-Shand in her personal stories from Zimbabwe:

> There was a belief that if a person greatly desired wealth—to succeed as a businessman for instance—and consulted a witchdoctor on how to achieve his goal, the *n'anga* would tell him to kill someone, take a specific organ (liver, heart, brain or genitals), and follow a set of instructions. If the person wanted to have a successful supermarket, he might be advised to hide the heart of a beautiful girl somewhere in the shop or under the foundation of the building; the spirit of the girl would attract customers to the shop. A person who intended to own a grinding mill might be advised to bury some brains near the mill, and so on. (Nzenza-Shand 1997:184–85)

During my interviews people frequently said that sorcerers "sacrifice" relatives for their own enrichment, meaning either literally killing or metaphorically neglecting them. Sometimes, when an *undofa* was involved, this was expressed through saying that these creatures demand to be fed meat: first, any meat, but later human flesh. Their hunger for flesh, however, is exceeded in popular belief by their thirst for blood. They can be vampires in a literal or a metaphorical sense, draining life from their victims. Drinking blood—in other words robbing the body of its life-force—is a common pattern in sorcery beliefs involving familiars. An elderly woman told me the following story, which was reported in the local media[5] in 1999 and caused tremendous concern among Bulawayo residents:

> Yes, perhaps the *ondofa* are responsible for AIDS. In the year 2000 [*sic*] there was a story in the news about frogs that drink blood from people. One of the sorcerers owning such frogs has even bought groceries for a willing victim. The frog was then bound to the victim's breasts and when it had finished feeding on her the sorcerer called a taxi and told the driver to drop this person at a certain place. The victim was no longer able to talk. She stayed somewhere in the neighboring township. He told her to "rest in peace" and that the money which she was given would be used at her funeral.

The frog was seen as a familiar owned by a sorcerer. The frog, like the *undofa*, was believed to grow out of a "root" and to mysteriously enrich its owner. The frog, like any familiar, benefited its owner by sacrificing someone else, a common pattern in sorcery beliefs, in this case by draining blood, the life-force, from the victim. Through such accounts the sorcerers' *ondofa* are blamed for all kinds of misfortunes and ailments in the neighborhood, including death. Once owners and their families have an *undofa*, the familiar will be with them permanently.

Some resort to home remedies designed to prevent the familiar from even approaching the house. These same remedies are used by people who want to prevent others' *ondofa* from harming them. I was told that the *ondofa* do not like salt; when they step on salt or taste it, they quickly run away. Sprinkling Holy Water, water blessed in various churches, is another remedy. However, most residents disagreed that it is so easy, saying it is necessary to employ experts, Christian exorcists or traditional healers, to get rid of them.

A bishop of an Apostle church explained to me how he deals with the creatures. If he wants merely to chase them away, he prays over water mixed with salt and sprinkles it throughout the house of the troubled person. When the creature realizes what the exorcist has done, it runs away. The bishop also lays traps, mainly of consecrated water. When he has caught an *undofa* he simply kills it, though he was reluctant to describe how he does it.

In this sense, the *undofa* differs from other spirit beings in the anthropological literature. The typical spirit can be driven out but not killed; it is immortal. The *undofa*, by contrast, has physical characteristics and therefore can be killed. Some members of Apostle churches even organize witch hunts in particular areas where sorcery is thought to be rampant, to rid the area of sorcerers and their familiars—including the *ondofa*.

The promiscuity of these creatures is a frequently mentioned characteristic that is relevant for understanding the interpretation of HIV/AIDS in terms of sorcery. Not surprisingly, the familiars' genitalia are extraordinarily large. Beliefs in both physical and non-physical beings that have non-consensual sexual relations with humans are observed cross-culturally.[6] Generally, the *ondofa* are thought to look for sexual partners outside the home of their owners. It becomes increasingly difficult, even dangerous, for the *ondofa*'s human sexual partners to fulfill their marital obligations with their spouses:

> The male *ondofa* want wives and will chase women's husbands away.
> If they are female, they want husbands, and they will chase the wives
> away when they want to sleep with their husbands. When these wives
> want to sleep with their husbands they would have to do so during
> the day, when it is light. At this time the *ondofa* will not interfere.

Women suffering due to the presence of these creatures are advised by local experts, who are knowledgeable in sorcery phenomena, to contact the creature's master. This is obviously difficult due to the secrecy of such practices.

The fact that marital relations, particularly sexual relations between spouses, are strained adds an interesting facet to the *undofa* belief. This belief spread with the movement of individuals across southern Africa, particularly through labor migration.[7] The *ondofa* are part of the South

African Xhosa tradition, which has been adopted by other ethnic groups in southern Africa. People told me that the "roots" used to "grow" an *undofa* come from South Africa, where many Zimbabweans go for work.

The diffusion of the *undofa* belief is made relatively easy in southern Africa due to the existence of comparable beliefs in familiars (Ngubane 1976:328). The *undofa*, with its exaggerated sexual features, exists in the context of labor migration, which heightened suspicions of marital infidelity. Such suspicions are common when there is long-term separation of spouses (Niehaus 2001:61). The sexually overactive *undofa* may be interpreted as a metaphor for the destructive side-effects of labor migration: marital infidelity and promiscuity.

This interpretation does not readily explain other sexual preferences of the creatures. They are also fond of young, unmarried girls, be they the owner's own daughters or the daughters of neighbors. The *undofa* thus represents not only suspicions of marital infidelity but also suspicions of premarital sex in a young woman. The *ondofa* can force any girl in the neighborhood to have sex. However, the owners have a role to play in this issue. They keep an *undofa* in order to accumulate wealth; in turn, they need to give something to the creature. Beyond shelter and food, this may include a sexual companion from among the owner's children or the children of others. A child is sacrificed for the personal gains of the sorcerer, a common aspect of sorcery practices. The girl is permanently damaged by the *undofa* because she is then unmarriageable.

People are usually not fully conscious during sexual encounters with *ondofa*, and only conclude that it took place after the event. Indicators are certain dreams and nightmares, as well as the presence of body fluids in the morning. The non-consensual manner of the acts is typical of sorcery beliefs. Zimbabweans are aware of other sorcery poisons that share some features with the *undofa* complex. These practices allow someone to have intercourse with women without their being aware of it (Feldskov and Frederiksen 2000:23; Mutandwa 1996). Women do not agree to the sexual advances but are taken unaware. The problem does not stop there, as the following statement of a healer shows:

> The *ondofa* make women "dirty," especially the uterus, and if the women are pregnant they give birth prematurely. When an *undofa*

has affected the female uterus we are able to correct it with traditional medicine. With the help of the medicines a lot of dirt comes out of the uterus. This is what is harmful to men, because this dirt enters the men during sexual intercourse and does not come out of them again. It will weaken the men who then have no energy any more.

In southern Africa, the belief is common that during sexual intercourse body fluids are mutually exchanged. Not only does male semen enter the female body but female body fluids are also absorbed by the male body. Informants maintain that the body fluids of one sexual partner even get sucked into the body of the other partner. If a married couple has sexual intercourse this does not represent a danger; oversimplified we could say that their bodies and fluids are "used to each other." However, when unmarried individuals have sex together, the act contaminates them and may result in some sort of health problem.

When this contamination is due to an *undofa*, it is even more serious. The *undofa*'s body fluids are stored inside the woman and she passes it on to all with whom she has subsequent intimate relations. This understanding of the sexual act has strong moral notions exhorting people not to have sexual relations outside marriage. Thus, I would argue that the risky exchange of body fluids is more a metaphor of morality than a local explanation of actual processes happening during sexual intercourse. Many people with whom I spoke, however, strongly believe in the factual truth of this understanding.

People believed that the sexually active *ondofa*, who harm others, were implicated in the AIDS epidemic. Research shows similar beliefs elsewhere in the region (e.g., Anderson 2002:427). Some interviewees, comparing the symptoms of *ondofa* abuse to AIDS symptoms, came to the conclusion that what biomedicine describes as AIDS is a condition caused by *ondofa* abuse. They regarded the *ondofa* as types of vampires feeding on people's blood. As the amount of blood in the body of victims decreases, the individuals become weaker and exhibit symptoms that are similar to those of AIDS, but are not AIDS-related:

The *ondofa* are killing others by drinking their blood. Their victims get thinner and thinner until they are only skin and bones. Then people will tell the sick that they have AIDS—but it is not AIDS, because their hair still has a healthy shine. These people are ill because an *undofa* is drinking blood from them. When such an individual goes to the Apostles to be prayed over in order to get healthy again, the Apostles will tell the person that the cause is an evil spirit. However, it is an *undofa* that is secretly doing these things. When the person goes to the clinic or hospital, the doctors will tell the person that the condition is caused by TB or AIDS, but this is a wrong diagnosis too.

According to informants, the symptoms of being abused by an *undofa* strongly resemble AIDS-related ailments: feeling weak, losing weight, and becoming increasingly emaciated. Many people argued that medical professionals incorrectly diagnose the victim's symptoms as caused by HIV/AIDS. Even the Apostles, leaders of indigenous churches, may wrongly interpret the symptoms in terms of spirit possession, which causes similar symptoms to HIV/AIDS, and as the abuse by *ondofa*. People carefully interpret and compare symptoms. The last quote shows that the interviewee was fully aware of the symptoms of full-blown AIDS, but identified other symptoms, such as healthy looking hair, that discredited the diagnosis of AIDS, TB, or even possession by a spirit. Some informants also argued that the fact that AIDS-related illness recurs is proof that it is caused by the *ondofa*:

> Long ago there were some sexually transmitted diseases. When you suffered from an STD you took medicine to cure it. Today, whatever you are given does not help. Even the most expensive medicine is ineffective, because the symptoms have a different cause; an *undofa* is killing you. The cause is not AIDS; the cause is the *undofa*.

In other words, if the symptoms were due to a regular disease, it would be possible to cure the patient. As mentioned earlier, recurring and persisting ailments are cross-culturally believed to be due to sorcery. It is not surprising, then, that HIV/AIDS becomes interpreted within the sorcery paradigm.

Other respondents believed that the *ondofa* are able to cause AIDS through sexual intercourse with humans. A study from west-central Zimbabwe concurs (Feldskov and Frederiksen 2000:23). People draw upon the traditional notion of pollution, which readily feeds into perceptions of pollution through sexual intercourse. The *ondofa* infect their male or female victims with HIV, polluting them with the virus by the same mechanism through which they have been polluting their victims before HIV reached southern Africa.

Infection with HIV through the *ondofa* is, however, only possible if some sort of physical nature is attributed to the *ondofa*. Other informants thought of them as non-physical beings that are just a preternatural outcome of sorcery poison. A traditional healer told me he is convinced that the *ondofa* cannot transmit HIV because they are merely non-material products of sorcery; they are not really living human beings. They can cause all kinds of harm, but not AIDS. He told me that, although they are thought to sleep with women, they do so only as figments of their imagination, which arises from sorcery. In other words, sexual intercourse is not really happening. This question, however, engendered lively debate:

> What I know about the *undofa* is that it is a kind of human being, or
> a kind of medicine that makes, out of something, a living human be-
> ing. If it is just a medicine that creates the being, then I do not believe
> it can spread AIDS. But if the *undofa* is really a "human" being, then
> I can imagine that sometimes it does spread AIDS. But if it is just a
> medicine, then I am not convinced that it can do so. I wonder if it has
> blood to do so.

The core of the discussion—that is, whether sexual intercourse with these creatures can transmit HIV or not—revolves around the question of whether they are bodily creatures with blood, or whether they are only magical poisons, the result of sorcery "medicines." The reference to blood points in the same direction. "Blood," however, refers in local languages in southern Africa not just to blood in the Western sense. It can also refer to semen. If this was implied by informants, then the argument has another subtle facet: the question is not only if the *ondofa* are material living beings or just imaginations triggered by sorcery, but if the creatures can actually produce semen (that is, engage in sexual intercourse with humans). They could be material beings, but incapable of having sex with humans.

In other accounts, a different line of thought became apparent. During discussions I was told that the *ondofa* have nothing to do with the AIDS epidemic. AIDS is only caused by those who are HIV-positive and deliberately infect others. They hide their evil intentions by blaming the *ondofa* for the AIDS epidemic. The following interviewee concurs:

> The ones who are HIV-positive, they are the ones who tell these lies that *ondofa* can give you AIDS.

As with the argument that sorcery accusations are a cover-up for a shameful disease, some Zimbabweans maintain that the *ondofa* are used to deflect attention from HIV/AIDS, which is associated with illicit and immoral sex. The physical suffering is attributed by sufferers to the presence of a familiar and thus not shameful. Residents who expressed such views to me strongly believe that HIV/AIDS is transmitted through sexual intercourse and not through sorcery.

Other people question the belief that HIV/AIDS is related to the *ondofa* by comparing the number of AIDS-related deaths with the assumed number of *ondofa* owned by sorcerers:

> Yes, you could believe that the *ondofa* infect you with AIDS. It is possible, but how many people have these *ondofa*! There may be one or two who have them. But not all people die because of them. I do not believe that they are responsible for so many AIDS deaths.

Such arguments did not cast doubt on the existence of *ondofa*, but rather on their being implicated in the AIDS epidemic. The *ondofa* are few and cannot be blamed for the high number of AIDS sufferers in the township. Instead of arguing that the high numbers of individuals suffering AIDS-related symptoms are a result of an "epidemic" of *ondofa*,[8] people argue that the few *ondofa* cannot possibly be held responsible for the widespread AIDS epidemic.

Notes

1. See, e.g., Bailey 1994:74–82; Glass-Coffin 1991:38; Kilpatrick 1997:4; Lewis 1970:304; Lussi 2002; and Merkur 1989:14.

2. The following are key studies on the question of "producing" a familiar by using another, even deceased, life form: Ashforth 2000:188–89; Berglund 1976:279; Crawford 1967:118–19; Darling 1999:735; Kaetzler 2001:90; Krige 1936:354–55; and Turner 1968:15.

3. Various publications present evidence, e.g., Berglund 1976:280–81; Kaetzler 2001:58–59; and Niehaus 2001:50–51.

4. See, for instance, Ardener 1970:147–57; Hoebel 1952:388; and Sanders and West 2003:167.

5. This incident is reported in Schoormann 2005:6–7.

6. See, e.g., Berglund 1989:117; Conco 1979:63; Pócs 1999:63; and Saler 1964:312.

7. Cross-culturally, the movement of people is associated with the dissemination of beliefs and practices (Evans-Pritchard 1929:637–38).

8. Ashforth (2002) argues that the large number of people suffering of full-blown AIDS results in an epidemic of witchcraft suspicions.

CHAPTER 5

Infidelity and Sorcery

Various informants explained the AIDS epidemic by referring to two common sorcery beliefs: *isidliso* and *ulunyoka*. The first is the generic term for a variety of poisons, known in southern Africa, which are added to either food or drink and taken by the unwitting victim.[1] Its name expresses this clearly: the verb *ukudla*, "to eat," with the suffix *isa*, "to make someone do," forms the verb *ukudlisa*, "to make someone eat," that is the root for this noun.[2] The second belief, *ulunyoka*, becomes operational after the victim touches items "doctored" with appropriate poisons.[3] These beliefs typically lead to the concocting of love potions.

Love potions[4] have a surprisingly wide distribution and serve a wide range of functions cross-culturally. Most frequently mentioned are bringing lost lovers back, inducing or destroying amorous feelings, undermining victims' control over their emotions, and inducing impotence or epileptic fits during sexual intercourse. Studies indicate that sorcery beliefs are highly diverse and even contradictory. The ways people have of putting ideas together outrun any neat distinction (Stewart and Strathern 2004:2).

Those who suspect their partners of sexual infidelity may try to influence their sexual behavior through *isidliso* and *ulunyoka*. People mentioned during interviews that marital relations are strained mainly by men's uncontrolled sexual behavior, and that men are more likely to engage in frequent sex with multiple partners than are women. Fearing their husbands' infidelity, women turn to *isidliso*:

> Some women use *isidliso* because they want to be loved by their husbands. They are afraid that their home is filling up [with children of their husbands by other women] and soon will be like a crowded township when the husband takes many wives! Therefore, they believe that it is better to use *isidliso*!

Women argue that the uncontrolled sexual behavior of men necessitates the use of such poisons. They fear that unfaithful husbands will impregnate other women and become responsible for the upbringing of their children. They also fear that their husbands will take several wives. Many women were highly critical of polygyny, pointing out the issue of jealousy among wives and the difficulty of being supported equally by the husband without favoritism. The purpose of *isidliso* is to direct the husband's attention solely toward his wife. In short, *isidliso* potions are seen as particularly useful when relationships are unstable or threatened (Keller 1978:497–99).

Despite such positive aims, *isidliso* is still a type of sorcery and thus regarded as improper and dangerous. People say *isidliso* is justified only when all other means of saving a marriage are exhausted. It is permissible to use it, as one old man told me, in order to *ukwakha umuzi* (build up the home), to strengthen the bond of marriage and protect the family. Several informants supported such a view:

> The purpose of *isidliso* is to put a fence around the home. Also, the women who trap their husbands do it to protect their homes by putting up a fence. This medicine is for protection and not for killing!

The use of *isidliso* can change a troublesome spouse into a domestic husband, a loving man submissive to his wife. He is "trapped" in his home and in the relationship with his wife, because the wife has through *isidliso* "put a fence" around the house making it impossible for him to look out for other women. Researchers report evidence of comparable beliefs and practices in other parts of the region and other countries.[5]

Though it is difficult to place diverse beliefs and practices neatly into clearly distinguishable categories, we can identify two types of *isidliso* love potions that women add to the food of their husbands. The first aims at positively influencing the behavior of men toward their wives. Some healers told me that wives frequently approached them asking for potions for several purposes: stimulating the love of an individual for them, preventing this person from falling in love with others, protecting such emotions from outside interference, and increasing his sexual desire and performance. Informants said that this use of *isidliso* has little relationship to the AIDS epidemic. However, they spoke of another use that is related to AIDS. Poisons are used for specific purposes: to lower the energy level of husbands, particularly their sex drive; to change roaming spouses into soft, calm stay-at-home husbands; and to keep husbands from spending time and money outside the home with other women (Chiroro et al. 2002:16–17).

While wives use *isidliso* to address infidelity, men do so by using *ulunyoka*. Many men are absent from their homes during the day, working either "downtown" or in the industrial areas of Bulawayo, or they may be outside the township looking for jobs. Following a long-established tradition of labor migration, a substantial number of Nkulumane male residents are away for prolonged periods of time working outside the country. Often a man could be away from home for weeks or months.

Currently, women too are increasingly forced by the harsh economic conditions in Zimbabwe to earn income for their families. Many engage in cross-border trading, necessitating prolonged absences from home. The fear of husbands that their wives may entertain men during the husbands' absence or during the women's absence from home is common. I was told that overly suspicious husbands even sweep the ground when they are leaving so they can identify footsteps of their wives' suitors when they return in the evening. One man said that the extent of wives' infidelity will only become evident when their contraceptives are taken away; then the number of unwanted pregnancies resulting from extramarital relations will skyrocket. A traditional chief voiced similar concerns some years ago in a local newspaper:

> The chief said the pill[6] was of major concern because most women who used it were becoming promiscuous. He said he preferred traditional methods of family planning [rather] than making the pill available to anyone who needed it. (Anonymous 1991b)

Modern contraceptives are easily accessible, allowing women to separate sex from conception. While men regard contraceptives as useful for family planning, they fear they will be used outside marriage. Such mistrust motivates some men to use a traditional poison with their wives to ensure their marital fidelity, namely *ulunyoka*; this potion is used only by husbands on their wives.

Informants describe three ways to administer *ulunyoka*. First, the poison can be secretly given to the wife by adding it to her food and drink. However, as men are generally not the ones preparing the meals, this is uncommon, more a confusion with *isidliso*. Second, a more commonly mentioned means of administering the substance is when the husband places an item treated with such poisons on the ground, hoping that his wife will walk over it. When she touches it, the poison will be operational. Third, the most commonly mentioned method is when the husband asks his wife to do something using an item treated with the poison. Informants said that for this purpose the husband uses a pocketknife, an item highly treasured by men in Zimbabwe. At times people mentioned padlocks. This use of a relatively modern item exemplifies the malleability of sorcery practices.

Along with traditional objects and practices, sorcerers take advantage of new things, as well as local methods. New technologies are easily drawn into inherited practices of sorcery (Romberg 2003:208, 257). Men use pocketknives and padlocks often, so they could easily have them doctored for sorcery without raising suspicion. These items have, however, a twofold symbolic meaning relevant for *ulunyoka*. This becomes evident in the following:

I have heard of the pocketknife that is prepared for this purpose. The husband carries it all the time. He leaves the pocketknife open. When his wife is unfaithful to him, the pocketknife will suddenly close! At that time she is sleeping with someone else.

This kind of *ulunyoka*, the one with the knife, serves the purpose to catch the two when they are still together and he still has an erection. This medicine causes them to continue their sexual encounter till the husband arrives.

When the sexual contact is initiated, and the knife automatically closes and magically locks the couple together, the two lovers cannot end their passion voluntarily (Gelfand 1967:151–54). They can only be released from their sexual encounter when the husband opens the pocket-knife again. In other words, this third type serves to alert the husband when his wife is having an extramarital affair and to give him the opportunity to catch them *flagrante delicto*. The cheated husband has sufficient proof of the misdoings of his wife, and takes immediate action. The husband knows that the poisons are already operational in his wife's adulterous lover, making him ill. Hoping for such results, men resolve to use *ulunyoka*:

It is said that a husband wants to use a sorcery poison on his wife so that she will be faithful to him. It is because he does not trust his wife! I know that a husband can trap his wife so that she is not sleeping around. And then he can go peacefully to work.

Both types of sorcery beliefs trigger fear in the minds of people, which serves to control their sexual behavior. While *isidliso* aims at enhancing male fidelity within marriage, *ulunyoka* functions to enhance female marital fidelity. Male residents in Nkulumane have reason to fear that the wives of other men could have been "doctored" with such poisons. This fear operates as a deterrent to engage in sexual relationships with them.

In other words, the mere suspicion that *ulunyoka* is used functions as a deterrent both for wives and for men courting them. *Isidliso* has a similar deterrent function. Husbands, fearing that their wives might refer to *isidliso,* control their sexual urges outside marriage so their wives will not feed them the potions. The two types of sorcery beliefs function, as do many sorcery beliefs, as a form of social control.

Other beliefs common in southern Africa serve this function. For example, a traditional belief posits that sexual encounters with married women result in physical ailments. An example is an account that appeared in a local newspaper saying that the promiscuous man sleeping with another man's wife gets sick [in this case, he gets cancer]:

> This reminds me of a good old-timer who always insisted that *ungath-andana lomfazi womuntu uzangenwa yimvukuzane.*[7] He always stressed that the infected person cannot be healed unless *uhlawule inkomo.*[8] Whether the old man's sentiments are true or not, it's neither here nor there, but one positive thing for certain is that it has helped to reduce infidelity among married couples as they fear to contract the deadly disease. And if more couples could be exposed to the old man's "gospel," then the spread of the HIV scourge would be greatly reduced. (Ncube 2003)

This belief discourages men from having sexual affairs with married women because, it promises, the pleasure of passion will be followed by a serious life-threatening disease.

The news report also referred to HIV/AIDS, arguing that this belief has a positive aspect: it motivates people to avoid sex with married women, thus preventing new HIV-infections. Women hoped that *isidliso* would have the same good effect. They expressed their fear during discussions that uncontrolled male sexual behavior endangers all of them. The following excerpt from an interview attests to this attitude:

> Our husbands are infecting us with AIDS; they go to many places, spoiling girls and the wives of others. At home we do not know about their sexual escapades. When they come home we just accept them as our husbands and sleep with them. We do not know what they have

done before they came home. Only they know. Now they are giving us this disease. We do not know how we can stay with our husbands. In the houses many are afraid of AIDS.

At times, woman informants portrayed the mens' assumed uncontrolled sexuality as even more drastic. Men's sexual prowess and greed cause them to continue searching for sexual encounters in times of sickness, including AIDS:

> When you see that your husband has this disease then it is better not to have sex with him anymore. But men who have AIDS often force themselves on their wives. The wives see the sores of their husbands and do not want to have sex with them. But the husbands still want to sleep with the wives and refuse to admit they are sick. If he is a strong man he will even fight with his wife and force her to sleep with him. It is like rape!

It appears that these frequent statements of women are not exaggerated. The tragic reality in Zimbabwe is that marriage has become the single biggest risk factor in HIV-infection for women because of their husbands' unprotected extramarital sexual encounters (Jackson 1999:139). A local poem expresses this sentiment, addressing marriage as we-die-together, as spouses giving each other the gift of death (Dube 2000). The subordination of women within marriage, their inability to address issues such as the promiscuity of their husbands and the use of condoms, and their material dependency on males expose women to this high risk (Farmer 1999:51; Makunike 2003).

Artist Shumba portrayed male/female sexual relations through a carving (page 94). The carving depicts a man who grabs a woman from behind, forcefully touching her and devouring her. The artist explained to me that the man represents a migrant laborer who came home after a long absence, having had sexual encounters with other women while he was away. His wife suspects that he has not been faithful to her, fears that he is HIV-positive, and refuses to have sex with him. So he takes her by force. He devours her, kills her. That is because he is HIV-positive.

Such portrayals of male sexual behavior, and the fear they imply,

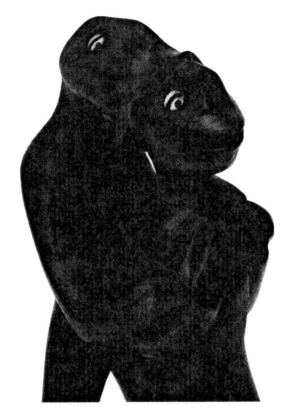

The migrant laborer. (Carving by Sheunesu Shumba. Photo by Heinz Helf.)

influence the local perception of the *isidliso* and *ulunyoka* poisons. Although the use of the poisons is generally viewed as immoral and illegal, some informants argued that the poisons are useful today in facing the AIDS epidemic. The poisons function as a strong deterrent to engaging in extramarital sex. People pointed out that this fear would not only reduce the number of extramarital affairs but also the incidents of HIV-infection. This corroborates what scholars argue about sorcery, namely, that it seeks to disarm the misfortunes of daily life (Bond and Ciekawy 2001:13; Devisch 2001:105). One middle-aged man told me about *ulunyoka*:

> AIDS is spread by those who go around and sleep with someone and then with someone else again. That is why in the old days they prepared *ulunyoka* so that he will not do so.

The local media report on the same function of *isidliso* by quoting a woman:

> In these days of AIDS you have to try by all means to keep one partner and ensure that he does not stray to other women, so these things are necessary. (Mlambo 1994)

The woman is referring to the use of *isidliso*, which prevents the husband from extramarital affairs, and thus protects both the husband and the wife from HIV.

A similar sentiment was expressed in a report in the local newspaper, which made headline news while I was conducting the study. It refers to the kind of *ulunyoka* that uses a padlock; however, in this case it is used by a wife to *khiya* (lock) her husband. This seems to be a new development, more akin to functions of *isidliso* or love potions. It is another example of the variability and malleability of sorcery practices.

The padlock has strong, self-explanatory symbolic meanings. The following report draws a connection to HIV/AIDS that can be applied to a form of *ulunyoka* in general:

Sources close to the faith healer said he may have helped "lock" hundreds of men. The fate of the men was unknown now that he has died. Some traditional healers interviewed said the victims "are now at the mercy of their wives" for good. . . . "My husband abandoned me and the children a few years ago for another woman. I was only saved by this other woman who advised me to approach Siziba for assistance. Siziba then asked me to buy a new padlock and a key, which he prayed for before locking it. . . . He actually saved my marriage. He 'locked' my husband and it did not take time before he came back to me and since then things have been normal in my family," said the woman, who works for a security company.

"When he came back, he never told me that he had problems performing in bed, but I could tell that Siziba's tricks had worked. When he started behaving, I eventually unlocked him and threw away the key, as I was worried that he might end up being impotent . . . ."

"If that is true, then we wonder how those people will live," said Thabani Ndlovu of Emakhandeni, "what will happen if the wife dies. The husband cannot remarry. To me that is witchcraft." A few years ago, Siziba admitted to *Chronicle* in an interview that he was indeed "locking" some husbands who were leaving their wives to enjoy themselves with girlfriends. "I just ask the woman to buy a padlock and bring it to me. The errant husband becomes a good family man instantly. I do this for the good of the nation. First, the spread of HIV/

AIDS is curtailed and second, it saves many families from breaking up," he was quoted then. (Chuma 2003)

The use of sorcery poisons to make husbands impotent when they attempt sexual relations with women other than their wives, or to negatively affect their fertility, is widely observed in southern Africa, including Zimbabwe (Keller 1978:501; Turner 1968:28). The healer's statement that he "locks" husbands because it is good for the nation facing HIV/AIDS is evidence of how such magical substances gained currency.

For many with whom I spoke, such sorcery practices serve as a deterrent against extramarital sexual relations and thus result in a reduction of HIV-infections. The same is said at times of HIV/AIDS itself. A short remark in a local newspaper exemplifies this:

I love ... AIDS for keeping partners faithful. (Anonymous 1991f)

The author of this statement sarcastically states that HIV/AIDS has a positive aspect, namely, the strengthening of marital fidelity because of the fear of acquiring HIV through extramarital relations. The fact that HIV continues to spread in Zimbabwe shows that fear is not a major factor in influencing human sexual behavior. The fear of contracting HIV does not appear to deter people from engaging in behavior with a high risk of getting infected. The fear of sorcery poisons is not a major deterrent either.

Though I use "poison" to refer to these practices, the question whether the poisonous nature of *isidliso* and *ulunyoka* is responsible for the intended outcome is not easily answered. The efficacy of these poisons is, according to informants as well as the literature, not solely determined by their ingredients. Sorcery poisons are believed to be operational both due to their magical character and to the poisonous nature of the substance. Some informants cited only the magical efficacy of the potions. These poisons cannot be understood in terms of modern toxicology because the poison is directed toward a particular individual.

Most people with whom I talked agreed that they are only operational with the individual for whom they were intended (Ashforth 2000:187). Another person can eat food contaminated with *isidliso* but not fall ill. The husband can have sex with his wife without being affected by *ulunyoka*. However, others emphasized the poisonous nature of the substances, especially *isidliso*, and believed that accidental wrong dosages can cause unintended results. Most people oscillate between the two perspectives without attempting to delineate them clearly.

These poisons can have serious side effects. The local media often take up this theme. Consider the following excerpt from a report about *isidliso*:

> However, what is interesting to note is that there are people who sleep during the day, not because they would have danced the night away or doing anything, they just feel sleepy. Some people believe that such people have been bewitched by their wives with a view of softening them. Usually these husbands are given the *muti*[9] who were harsh to their wives, who then think that the only way out of the problem is to make them eat the puppy eyes or anything (*ukudlisa*) that would make them softhearted. (Ndlovu 2003b)

The implicit message is that *isidliso* negatively impacts the health of the husband, making him weak and feeble. The aim may be greater than simply hurting his sexual performance with another woman. The serious effects of a high dose of wrongly administered poison may be fatal. Informants said that the death of the husband may be the goal of an irate wife. One elderly man pointed out various homes of wives who are said to have used such poisons to kill their husbands. All over Africa people are aware of the lethal use of such poisons.[10]

Fortunately for husbands, deliberate poisoning is rare; in most cases men are the household providers and murdering them would cause hardships for the wives. Keeping a troublesome husband alive is still the lesser evil for the wives! However, sometimes something goes terribly wrong and the husband becomes seriously ill and dies. Proof of sorcery poisoning is difficult due to the secretive nature of the practices and because symptoms of sorcery-induced ailments are similar to those of other (particularly chronic) conditions. To make sure that the cause of ill health is a sorcery poison, people need to consult experts, diviners or healers, who know how to interpret the symptoms.

The question is, what are the symptoms of the two types of sorcery poisons? Let us first look at *isidliso*. Traditional healers with whom I spoke concur with reports from other areas in southern Africa that, in the body, *isidliso* initially enters the lungs, stomach, or digestive tract, causing pain and various illnesses of these organs (Ashforth 2001a:9). Persistent pain in these organs indicates that the poison is now firmly entrenched. The person gets increasingly weaker, drained of energy. At this point the working of the *isidliso* substances is imagined as miniature animals that, like lizards, slowly eat away the inner parts of the victim. The poison slowly consumes its victim, causing persistent diarrhea and continuing weight loss. Mouth sores are another symptom that was frequently mentioned by my informants. All these symptoms lead to a slow wasting of the body. The increasing emaciation is usually expressed by saying *umzimba udliwe* (the body is eaten), either by mysterious beings created through *isidliso* or by the actual working of the poison. If the wife used an overdose of this poison, the husband dies in excruciating pain. Similar beliefs are evidenced across the region and have some relation to comparable beliefs from other regions of the globe.[11]

When *isidliso* is suspected, the victim must engage a powerful healer to remove it. In contrast to views from South Africa that most if not all healers can heal *isidliso* (Ashforth 2001a:10), Zimbabweans generally believe that only a few experts among the traditional healers and curers in indigenous churches are able to do so. The latter frequently replace the use of traditional medicines with prayer for healing. A traditional healer gave me a systematic account of how to cure it.

First, the poison has to be removed, otherwise it will kill the victim. When very strong medicines are used, the *isidliso* poisons are removed too quickly and leave bleeding wounds behind wherever they are attached (the stomach or lungs), resulting in the victim's death. Slow-working medicines have to be used first to gently remove the poisons and give the wounds time to heal. The second step is to induce diarrhea to rid the body of the poisons that are now detached and loose in the digestive tract.

The third and last step in this sequence is to strengthen the body through traditional medicines. A special diet may accompany this treatment.

Ulunyoka exhibits comparable patterns. Recall that it is a powerful destructive medicine for affecting the lover of the wife, who becomes ill and, if not treated properly, dies after a long illness. The sickness does not develop immediately, but over time. We can distinguish two types of *ulunyoka* according to the onset and duration of the sickness. In Zimbabwe, one type affects the wife's lover immediately following sexual intercourse, and a second type triggers the same results but with a delayed action—the lover's condition will slowly deteriorate and he will die within a year or so (Walters 1980). During my interviews I was only told about the second type.

We can also distinguish various types of *ulunyoka* according to the ingredients used, the symptoms caused by them, and the intended results.[12] Actually, the ingredients used for a particular poison explain the resulting symptoms and the intended outcome. For instance, pounded bees will cause pain in the wife's lover that is comparable to being stung by bees; using parts of a particular snake is believed to cause behavior resembling the movements of snakes due to unbearable stomach pain, as well as the peeling of the skin in the manner of snakes. Informants in Nkulumane concurred with the literature and described these symptoms in stark detail:

> The stomach starts swelling. The person, being in pain, moves on his stomach like a snake. I even saw it with my own eyes, and then the skin peels off the stomach! This kind of *ulunyoka* really works.

For some kinds of *ulunyoka*, genitals of dogs are used, which may be the reason that mutilated dogs are reported from time to time in the local media in Bulawayo (Anonymous 1991c; Zhakata 1992). Respondents in Nkulumane explained to me that the use of such ingredients is to make the wife and her lover so overcome by sexual passion—like mating dogs—that they forget all caution and do not separate until the husband of the woman discovers them *flagrante delicto*. The man does not lose his erection until the husband arrives. Canine sexual passion has the same symbolic meaning as the padlock and the pocketknife: locking the couple together.

In most interviews about *ulunyoka*, informants argued that persistent swelling of the abdomen and excruciating pain are the most common signs that a man has had sexual intercourse with a woman "doctored" by her husband with *ulunyoka*. This symptom has been portrayed in another of Shumba's carvings (below). Other symptoms include diarrhea alternating with severe constipation, as well as continual dry cough, skin eruptions, and tremors, coupled with other symptoms such as weight loss and extreme weakness.[13] These symptoms vary according to the poison used but have in common that the patient will die unless treated by traditional means (Munk 1997:10). The following is an example from my interviews:

> When a man's stomach becomes swollen because of *ulunyoka*, his relatives ask him, if he has been sleeping with someone's wife. If he has courage he will admit it and ask his relatives to go to the husband of the woman and start discussing the fine he should pay. If they come to an agreement quickly, before the poison severely damages him, he will soon get better, because the one who gave him *ulunyoka* released him from that condition. It is like being caught by the police. When you agree to pay the fine (for example, some heads of cattle), then you will be given the antidote. I remember one man from Lupane. He had his own wife, but he was having sex with women of other men. He became sick, it was said, because of *ulunyoka*. This man was affected by *ulunyoka*; his stomach was terribly swollen and it was very painful for him. The hospital

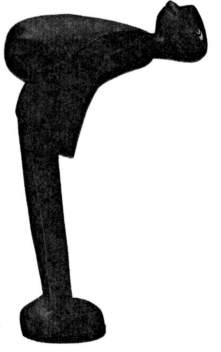

Ulunyoka. (Carving by Sheunesu Shumba. Photo by Heinz Helf.)

tried to treat him but nothing helped. Only the *ulunyoka*-antidote, given to him by the husband of the woman with whom he had slept, would have saved him. But this husband wanted him to die. Perhaps he was afraid that if he gives him the antidote that he will do it again.

Expressing suspicions of sorcery publicly can be dangerous. Accusing someone of being a sorcerer may even become a matter for the courts. For this reason, sorcery suspicions are well-kept secrets within the family. However, initiating a process of investigation is crucial for successful treatment. To determine if *ulunyoka* had been used, a sick man first has to reveal that he slept with a married woman; then her husband can be approached, presented with an apology, and with a request for an antidote (the appropriate traditional medicine for curing the condition).

Understandably, men are reluctant to express their suspicion that they are victims of sorcery. They could try to contact directly a local expert knowledgeable in treating *ulunyoka* poisons. However, the surest way to get healed is to get the antidote prepared by the same expert who gave the *ulunyoka* poisons to the husband to "lock" his wife. Without the appropriate medicinal substances to treat the condition, the *ulunyoka* victim continues to suffer excruciating pain, becomes increasingly emaciated, and finally dies.

The *isidliso* and *ulunyoka* complex has been appropriated as a vehicle for explaining HIV/AIDS in Zimbabwe, elsewhere in southern Africa, and in other parts of the world.[14] The frequently mentioned loss of energy, the slow wasting of the body, and the two poisons' effect on the breathing and digestive systems of the victim strongly resemble AIDS-related symptoms. Further, there are moral parallels that people draw between the two diseases: both are seen within a context of immoral sexual relations (Scott and Mercer 1994:86–87). Because of these similarities, it comes as no surprise that some Zimbabweans drew the conclusion that HIV/AIDS is not a new disease but actually the result of using *isidliso* and *ulunyoka* poisons.[15]

Such views have been challenged. For example, a comment in the question/answer section of a local newspaper from the early years of the epidemic clearly disputes an association of HIV/AIDS with *ulunyoka*:

> *Question:* AIDS is a disease caused by a spell on an unfaithful woman by her jealous partner. Beer-hall gossip?
> *Answer:* Definite beer-hall gossip! AIDS is spread through sex with infected persons. (Anonymous 1990a)

People with whom I spoke also raised doubts about a connection of *isidliso* or *ulunyoka* with HIV/AIDS. Despite the close resemblance in symptoms, they argued that the conditions are distinct. They maintained that, for example, *isidliso* would only affect its intended victim—for instance, the husband when the poison is administered by the wife. They argue too that *ulunyoka* affects only the wife's lover. The wife herself is unharmed, and her ailing lover does not transmit the ailment to others. In contrast, HIV/AIDS affects both spouses and, at times, even their children. This pattern of infection indicates that it is unlikely that any kind of sorcery is at work. Sorcery usually affects only the intended victim.

Another argument against the interpretation of AIDS as *isidliso* is that frequently those affected are young people who are not likely to be victims of the poisons. Residents observed that children and adolescents, as well as unmarried adults, at times exhibit symptoms that could be *isidliso*. This age group would not yet be in the relationships with spouses where poison is generally thought to be used. To some degree this argument also applies to *ulunyoka*. Because this poison is mainly used by husbands to "lock" their wives, unmarried adolescents who had sexual intercourse only among themselves and who exhibited such symptoms would be unlikely victims of this type of sorcery.

Consequently, some people rejected the interpretation of HIV/AIDS in terms of *ulunyoka* or *isidliso*. They argued that the phenomena are clearly distinguishable and that AIDS is an illness different from those ailments caused by sorcery. Some even argued that referring to *isidliso* and *ulunyoka* is just a strategy to deviate attention from a stigmatized and socially unacceptable disease to a phenomenon which is not only culturally acceptable but which also points at others as culprits. Consider the following:

Only a few openly admit that someone has AIDS. Often it is said that such a person was bewitched or given *isidliso*. They say that one is bewitched, although they see symptoms that cannot be due to *isidliso*. It is difficult for a parent in particular to accept that the child has this disease. Therefore, they say that their child has been given *isidliso*. Perhaps "slow poison"[16] was added to his food. Perhaps the relatives are responsible for it, or the wife if the husband is sick. The wife has made him sick.

This underscores what was argued earlier, namely that sorcery suspicions are sometimes just a cover-up hiding a shameful and stigmatized disease. Unsuccessful treatment within the sorcery paradigm through traditional healers will reveal the truth, that the sickness was AIDS. *Isidliso* and *ulunyoka* are curable, while AIDS is not (Anonymous 1991a).

Notes

1. Also, in other parts of the world, women were found to practice sorcery through food. See, for example, Aguirre Beltrán 1980:227; Behar 1987:40; Hove 1985:107; Sahagún 1981:150–51; and Cirac Estopañán 1942:81–83.

2. Other regional languages have terms for such poisons with a comparable meaning. See, e.g., Ashforth 2005:9; Schapera 1970:113–14; and Schoormann 2005:360.

3. *Ulunyoka* is associated with the Tonga and other people living in the Binga or Gokwe area of southern Zimbabwe and southern Zambia, and is widely known in southern Africa. The Tonga people have the reputation of being powerful sorcerers, both in my interviews and in the literature, as reported, e.g., by Keller 1978:491; McGregor 1999:138; Schoormann 2005; and Simmons 2002:381. The wide distribution of variants of *ulunyoka* is reported, e.g., Conco 1979:62, 69; Feldskov and Frederiksen 2000:26; Jackson 1988:102, 107; Munk 1997:10; and Niehaus 2001.

4. From the rich literature on the cross-cultural use of love potions, see, e.g., Behar 1987:36–38; Bonner 1950:115; Bowden 1987:190; De Mello e Souza 2003:142–52; Freyre 1966:333; Galt 1991:741–42; Gijswijt-Hofstra 1999:176; Gentilcore 1992:211; Golomb 1993:42; Gordon 1999:194; Hastrup 1990:233–35; Leclerc-Madlala 2001:543; Michelet 1995:89–97; Ogden 1999:35; Percival and Patel n.d.:13; Rodman 1979:28; Schrauwers 2003:133–38; Siegel 2003:141; Sweet 2003:173; and Wittman 1933:65.

5. For example, Behar 1987:40–43; Gentilcore 1992:215; Gordon 1999:196–97; Keller 1978:500–501; and Lewis 1961:141.

6. The pill refers to the most common form of contraception, as tablets.

7. This literally means "if you love the wife of someone else, then you will contract cancer."

8. The phrase means that the culprit has to "compensate by paying a fine of cattle."

9. *Muti* is the anglicized form of *umuthi*.

10. See, e.g., Ashforth 2002:121–22; Gordon 1999:197; Ingstad 1989:250.

11. See, e.g., Ashforth 2002:129–30; Darling 1999:738; Loeb 1929:82; Park 1934:110; Pollock 1996:329; Salamon 1983:415–16; and Walker 1989:5.

12. Distinguishing different types of *ulunyoka* according to symptoms is reported, e.g., by Gelfand 1967:151–54; 1985:231; Hutchings et al. 1996:306; Niehaus 2001:103, 219; and Zhakata 1992.

13. Medical doctors argue that *ulunyoka* becomes a blanket explanation for prostate problems, bilharzias, epididymo-orchitis, intestinal and abdominal ailments, schistosomiasis, renal failure, STDs, hepatitis B, and other illnesses. See, e.g., Conco 1979:62; and Jackson 1988:102.

14. This has been argued, e.g., by Ashforth 2000:167, 2002:121–22; Kroeger 2003:245–48; Marcus 2002:90; and Wolf 1996a:154.

15. Regarding *isidliso* see, e.g., Schmitt 1999:86. For *ulunyoka* see local newspaper reports (e.g., Munyavi 1990) and novels (e.g., Kala 1994:7)

16. This English phrase is sometimes used to denote *isidliso*, because it is believed to affect a person only slowly over time.

PART III

HIV/AIDS and Conspiracy

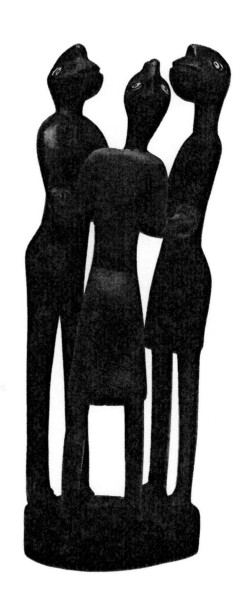

CHAPTER 6

Conspiracy Paradigms

The AIDS epidemic became anchored in another thought pattern familiar to people: conspiracy suspicions. Scholars from various disciplines define conspiracy theories as attempts to explain the cause of an event as a secret, deceptive plot by a covert alliance. *Conspiracy theory* as a term carries a negative connotation, because conspiracy fears generally lack sufficient verifiable evidence to be taken seriously.

Conspiracy theories interpreting the origin of AIDS as the outcome of an insidious plot have circulated all over the world within diverse social groups in both scientific and popular sectors since AIDS entered the public consciousness. Academics have used at least two different approaches to explain this phenomenon: first, by looking into the deeper conflicts that reside in the psyche,[1] and second, by studying the conflicts in a society.[2] Research indicates the two approaches can be investigated separately, but must be seen together because the sociological contexts and psychological processes are interrelated (Kramer 1994:223). I mention both approaches in order to highlight the variegated and complex meanings of AIDS conspiracy fears.

Where did AIDS come from? I heard this question frequently in Zimbabwe. Conspiracy theories offer answers to the questions of the origin of the disease, whether there is an agent, who the agent is, if there is a mastermind and, if so, who it is. As such, conspiracy theories belong to a broad, cross-cultural category of origin narratives. Etiological stories form a significant part of most folklore collections, providing narrative explanations for such issues as how we came to our current state of being and how the things that we take to be normative developed. AIDS narratives are no different. AIDS conspiracy fears reveal people's concern with origins, with establishing a source for the disease. Knowing the origin establishes some intellectual control over it and helps in formulating prevention strategies (Goldstein 2004:77–78; Waldby et al. 2005:11). Conspiracy theories, like sorcery beliefs, are fundamentally defense mechanisms that help people cope with insecurity, alleviate anxiety, and give hope that the wheel of misfortune can be turned around.[3] A related question that conspiracy suspicions, like sorcery beliefs, try to answer is: Why has this happened to me (I am basically a good person) or to my society, which is virtuous?[4] People tend to personalize the cause for their misfortune by attributing blame to malevolent agents, which are usually some sort of "outsider" or "other."[5] As such they are examples of scapegoating constructions and other persecutory belief systems (Kruglanski 1987:219; Taylor 1992:62).

The problem with knowing the origin of HIV is, to some extent, its lack of credible knowledge. Since the beginning of the AIDS epidemic, controversies regarding the origin of HIV have been common within academia. Some scientists expressed their doubts regarding the etiology of HIV:

> It seems strange that so many primate-to-human lentivirus transfers have occurred in recent history. (Weiss 2003:S11)

The dissemination of such statements by scientists quickly raised questions outside academia that something is at work that is at best mysterious and at worst a malicious plot.

Zimbabweans told me they were aware of the controversy surrounding the origin of HIV/AIDS, including the conspiracy suspicions. They said that most of what they know about the genesis of the virus is just hearsay, gossip, or rumor, and that the actual truth is not known. A middle-aged man summarized what many people thought:

> There are so many theories on the origin of AIDS. Speaking about the origin of HIV/AIDS is just a kind of debating and we do not know the truth. I do not believe such theories, because we have no proof. We really do not know where the virus came from.

Local poems reflect this general view that the origin of HIV is unknown and go even further. Debates about the genesis of the epidemic lead to the reciprocal attribution of blame, with Africans blaming Westerners and Westerners blaming Africans (e.g., Mabuya 1998). I observed this during my fieldwork. The origin of the disease is not known, yet people engaged in lively discussions about it. Lack of knowledge has rarely stopped conspiracy theories. Conspiracy suspicions, very much like sorcery suspicions, seem to flourish in a shadow of doubt surrounding empirical evidence for a threatening event.[6]

Lack of knowledge certainly did not stop some Nkulumane residents from looking for answers and constructing their own theories about the origins of HIV. Such processes are motivated, like sorcery beliefs, by a suspicion that there is more happening than meets the eye—invisible powers are at work, shaping the fortune of others. Our everyday world is simply a facade that masks a deeper, more important, and [more profound reality,] one that lies beyond our immediate comprehension (Ashforth 1996:1220; Todd 2003:160).

In this perception, Zimbabweans do not stand alone. Speculation about the origins and modes of transmission of HIV/AIDS is shared through rumor and gossip in many countries. Though the processes have similar patterns, the actual conspiracy theories being created and disseminated take on new motifs, new elaborations, and new concerns—and sometimes develop into entirely different narratives.[7]

In Zimbabwe, rumor about AIDS sometimes surfaced in public discussions. I took part in a workshop on HIV/AIDS awareness at the Roman

Catholic Church in Plumtree that was conducted by a nurse from the Umzingwane AIDS Council and attended by about thirty community leaders from the surrounding rural areas. This workshop is an example of people's curiosity about the origin and genesis of HIV/AIDS, so typical of what I encountered on numerous occasions in Bulawayo.

The participants of the workshop listened attentively when the nurse first spoke about various sexually transmitted diseases, their symptoms, and their treatment. She explained that HIV/AIDS is incurable, and described how HIV is contracted, and how to protect oneself from infection. She identified HIV/AIDS as a sexually transmitted disease and cited the individual's behavior as the ultimate factor responsible for acquiring the virus. For protection she referred to the "ABC" method: "abstain, be faithful, and use a condom," widely disseminated in Africa (Green 2003, Green and Herling 2006). Some participants were worried by what the nurse said. Finally one man spoke up:

> We appreciate and accept what you present to us today about the
> AIDS epidemic. However, there is still an important issue left out—the
> question why this disease is such an immense problem. I want to ask
> the question where this illness comes from and who was instrumental
> in bringing it to us! If we do not shed light on this question, then our
> efforts to tackle the disease will be futile.

The nurse repeated the biomedical explanation of HIV transmission, adding that AIDS is a sexually transmitted disease that must be taken seriously and other knowledge about the epidemic is irrelevant. She told the participants that we do not know where HIV/AIDS originated or if someone was instrumental in its origin. Her position was in line with what most medical personnel told me, as seen in publications of those working in the field of HIV prevention in Zimbabwe and beyond (Loewenson and Whiteside 1997:5; Duh 1991:60).

The head of Uganda's AIDS committee commented metaphorically: "There is a snake in the house. Do you just sit and ask where the snake came from?" Some political leaders express the same view. Kenneth Kaunda, when he was still president of Zambia, asserted in 1987: "What is more important than knowing where the disease came from is knowing

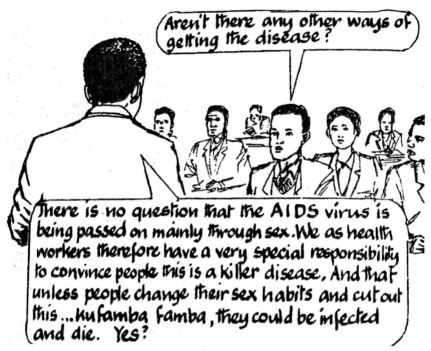

Questioning the explanation that HIV/AIDS is a sexually transmitted disease. *Kufamba famba* is a Shona term meaning to "move around," with connotations of sexual promiscuity. (Anonymous, 1990d)

where it is going."[8] Many African leaders and healthcare workers thought inquiring into the issue of HIV origins to be futile and a waste of time. For them it was more important to focus on knowledge about the disease per se and how to prevent infection. A similar pattern is portrayed in a Zimbabwean instructional leaflet dealing with the causes of the AIDS epidemic (above). However, avoiding this question satisfied neither the participants of the workshop in Plumtree nor the residents in Nkulumane. For them, the question of the origin of the disease was crucial.

The importance given to the search for the origin of the AIDS epidemic is, to some extent, motivated by traditional healing systems. Investigating the underlying cause of illness is central to African and other non-Western healing systems.[9] Diverse strategies for identifying the causes of ill health are known in various parts of the continent. The functions of such a search are succinctly summarized by du Toit:

> Ignorance of cause and effect leaves a person ineffective and once again increases anxiety. Knowing, on the other hand, what causes or threatens misfortune leads to a range of actions, some prophylactic, some precautionary, and some positive (du Toit 1985:164).

Thus, when one goes to a traditional healer looking for treatment for an ailment, the question of causality is of prime importance: Healers and diviners attempt to identify cause and origin in order to prescribe the proper and effective treatment. Such thought patterns are not only crucial in actual divination events but also pervade popular thinking. One informant gave the following example, which is based on a widespread narrative that HIV/AIDS originates from sexual intercourse with dogs. Believing it to be literally true, the individual argued that this knowledge could be an avenue to finding a cure:

> If it is true that the disease originates from an animal such as a dog, we need to observe dogs and what they do when they are sick. Is it not true that dogs, although they are carnivores, sometimes eat grass if their body requires it? Animals know how to treat themselves! If HIV/AIDS comes from a dog, then dogs might provide us with cues to find a cure for AIDS.

Others thought that HIV originated in primates and then somehow crossed over to humans:

> It is said that in the wilderness there are monkeys who do not get AIDS although they are infected with HIV. Scientists observed this and took blood from these monkeys and injected it into humans, attempting to immunize them. But the people died of AIDS, contrary to the monkeys, who do not develop full-blown AIDS because they live on wild foods.

It was thought that, by identifying the origin of the virus and the pathway through which the virus entered humans, and by observing the behavior of vectors through which HIV crossed over to humans, we could identify a cure for AIDS. If the vectors are animals, then we need to observe them carefully. If the vectors are malicious human agents, their identification may help to identify a cure. If someone evil is instrumental in the genesis of HIV/AIDS, then it is imperative to identify and to obtain information from this individual, thus, providing clues that could be helpful in the search for a treatment. The following is an example of such a view:

> It is a pity that we do not know who is responsible for AIDS. If we knew the person, then we could ask if that individual knows of a cure.

In other words, locating the origin of HIV and AIDS in human intentions means somehow to find a cure, an easy solution to all the problems that have followed the origin of HIV (Kruger 1996:251–52). These and similar responses, were however, accompanied by a problematic issue, namely that people showed little interest in finding out how a particular individual acquired HIV. The sexual transmission of HIV and how to prevent it was of secondary importance for people concerned with the origin of the virus. They focused on the origin and genesis of HIV, believing that such knowledge would aid in finding a cure. Their interest was in healing AIDS, not in preventing HIV-infection.

If the conspirators planned and carried out evil acts in the past, they are successfully active in the present, and will triumph in the future if those with information do not prevent their sinister doings. Scholars point out such a rationale underlies both conspiracy fears and sorcery suspicions. Research shows that determining who or what might be responsible for misfortune is necessary to afford protection against further mishap (Ashforth 2005:69; Kruglanski 1987:220). Informants explained that if there is an unidentified evil force behind the disease, then neither prevention nor cure will help. This agent will find another way to inflict harm. An elderly woman told me that evil agents causing epidemics is not a new problem:

It is not the first time that they do so. Long ago we were troubled by the Spanish influenza. Now they bring us AIDS.

There is historical evidence from Zimbabwe that people blamed the colonial administration for the Spanish influenza of 1918–1919 (Shelley 1918). The suspicion that epidemics, such as the Rinderpest of 1986, were introduced by an evil European agent is nothing new in southern Africa (van Onselen 1972:478). It is commonly believed that in more recent times the Rhodesian forces used viruses during the liberation war in order to counter the insurgency (McGregor 1999, White 2004). The fact that some residents in Nkulumane do not regard HIV/AIDS as an isolated single incident is important; for them the current epidemic is just a piece of a large puzzle of evil conspiracies and attempts to inflict harm on them. History reminds them that some malicious force tried to harm them before, a common pattern in conspiracy theories globally. This agent caused harm but did not succeed in total destruction. This force is trying again to harm them, now by using HIV/AIDS; it will not give up until it succeeds or is stopped. Such statements have a sense of urgency: identify the evil force behind HIV/AIDS before we are destroyed.

We can interpret Zimbabwean AIDS suspicions by referring to the societal context in which they emerged, an approach applied to conspiracies in the West.[10] Analysis of their patterns shed light on Zimbabwean conspiracy fears. Conspiracy beliefs worldwide, much like sorcery beliefs, identify potential enemies through an interpretation of the forces that negatively impact the life of the blamer (Farmer 1992:242–43; Niehaus and Jonssen 2005:201).

Conspiracy theories are prevalent in groups that have endured harmful assaults by outsiders. Experiencing discrimination, disempowerment, and other demeaning conditions helps to explain the formulation and acceptance of conspiracy theories.[11] Conspiracy theories across cultures, like sorcery beliefs, stem largely from a sense of diminished human agency, a feeling that individuals and groups are not able to control their own lives, and so suspect some sort of alien agency is secretly directing them.[12]

Also like sorcery beliefs, conspiracy fears grow out of views about how the world works.[13] They are grouped under the term *ethnosociology*, that is, theories ordinary people use to explain challenging social conditions (Waters 1997:114).

People's painful experiences do not contradict this type of causal explanation. The experiences are used by believers in conspiracies, such as Cantwell, Cress-Welsing, Gilbert and Porter as proof for their theories.[14] As conditions differ from society to society and from social group to social group, conspiratorial thinking may take on vastly different forms across the globe (Sanders and West 2003:5; Zonis and Joseph 1994:430).

The African American experience of maltreatment and deception by government feeds conspiratorial thought, including AIDS conspiracy fears (Hawkins 2005:26; Sobo 1995:44). Various scholars believe that the Tuskegee Experiment resulted in general mistrust of the medical profession and the government that contributed to the formulation of AIDS conspiracy theories among African Americans.[15] The U.S. Public Health Service conducted the Tuskegee project, involving some 600 African American men for forty years, ending in the early 1970s. During the study, treatment for syphilis was withheld from them in order to chart the "natural history of the disease." The legacy of this medical project goes far beyond the borders of the United States; through the mass media this study became known throughout the world, feeding suspicions of conspiracies in other locales, including Zimbabwe.

Recurring harmful experiences are, in Social Representations Theory, familiar patterns within which HIV/AIDS became anchored and acquired meaning. Identifying parallels with other social issues, believers in conspiracy theories concluded that the AIDS epidemic is another incident of neglect and even abuse by the dominant in society, who have caused hardship before.[16] These familiar patterns represent a so-called welcome structure through which misfortune is explained (Groh 1987:3, 2001:189). Again, as with sorcery suspicions, familiar patterns foster a tendency to become a closed system of ideas, which absorbs criticism and converts it to strengthen the claim.[17] Researchers looked for historical and other evidence to support suspicions. Chapters 7 and 8 show how such experiences shaped the evolution of Zimbabwean conspiracy suspicions.

People's desire to uncover the origin of HIV/AIDS in order to find a cure and to disarm the evil force that is inflicting harm on them is not really addressed by HIV/AIDS awareness and prevention campaigns. The mass media fill this void. They play an important role in health education in the developing world, where other sources of information about HIV/AIDS are not readily available.[18] The print media especially represent a source of information for township residents making sense out of the epidemic. A high literacy rate in Zimbabwe, and the availability and affordability of certain print media, particularly in urban areas, make print an important means of getting information. Zimbabweans use print media for information, while they use TV and radio mostly for entertainment. Generally, the families I knew were not paying much attention to what was said on the radio or TV but they read print media and shared news with their friends. Printed materials were thus the most important source of information for AIDS beliefs—even more influential than advice from medical personnel.[19]

The younger generation displayed print media to signal their sophistication; young men and women often carried a newspaper, a magazine, or an instructional leaflet. On weekends, many are seen with prayer books and hymnals on their way to church. Generally the individual carrying such materials is not the only one reading them. A single copy quickly moves from one person to another, and the worn condition of some monthly magazines indicates they had gone through many hands. The age of the publication is of secondary relevance; a magazine that was published several months ago is still shared with others. Even old newspapers are not discarded but read repeatedly. At times they are sold at the local flea market to be used for other purposes, such as wrapping vegetables, but buyers can be seen reading the outdated news stories.

This is important for understanding local AIDS beliefs; publications of several years ago can still influence contemporary perceptions of the epidemic. The date of publication is irrelevant; a published report is discussed and remembered, becoming a template for evolving theories, and quickly adapting to various local contexts (Pipes 1997:121; Treichler 1999:220).

The reliance on mass media for information about HIV/AIDS is highly problematic because it is not clear whether the source of the evidence is credible (Turner 1993:153). One goal of the popular media frequently is to grab attention. Erroneous beliefs may make better newspaper copy than scientifically correct facts (Bledsoe 1990:199). Thus, anecdotal reports of AIDS in the United States and Europe are often disseminated through the Zimbabwean press, while reports on the local AIDS situation take on a secondary role. The then-minister for Health and Child Welfare, physician Timothy Stamps, reacted to the disastrous potential of such news in Zimbabwe and even called for a ban in 1994 on erroneous reports in the press (Webb 1997:85). Some informants, critical of the accuracy and reliability of the mass media, were cautious when referring to media reports:

> I was shown a magazine at home. I think it was in 1972 [sic]. This magazine was *Parade*. It said in the magazine that AIDS threatens only blacks and was produced deliberately by whites. But when you read something like that, you cannot take it as absolute truth, because at times journalists tell us lies.

Although the interviewee did not remember the correct date, his reference in the same interview to the Non Aligned Movement summit, which was held in 1986 in Zimbabwe, clarified that he actually referred to an issue of *Parade* from 1986, seventeen years before the interview. During the summit, Zimbabwean and other print media reiterated the arguments that HIV/AIDS was a deliberate plot to harm blacks (e.g., Anonymous 1986). People were still, in 2003, aware of the arguments presented in the news years ago, but approached the information with caution, not trusting its source. People believe that journalists do not tell the truth.

The print media are a major source for Zimbabweans in formulating their own conspiracy theories. This is in contrast to sorcery beliefs, which appear to be less informed by the mass media; to a large degree, sorcery beliefs are triggered by preexisting traditional beliefs and practices. It is striking how closely conspiracy suspicions, presented in the mass media throughout the years, resemble those that I observed in the township during the course of my research. My observation supports the assertion that the mass media are the source of many conspiracy theories. Scholars argued the same for conspiracy fears elsewhere (Goldberg 2001:232–33).

The mass media, particularly the print media, are providing venues for discussing local conspiracy theories while adding some local flavor, especially in letters to the editor. Local theories in the township closely match those expressed in letters to the editor (e.g., Chimuchembere 1992; Nyikadzino 1991; Wadawareva 1992). Such letters have the following in common: First, that AIDS is a conspiracy tracing back to presumptive American racial attitudes against blacks. Second, an AIDS conspiracy is thought to be just one in a series of attacks on blacks. (Again examples from the United States are cited, such as the suspicion that African Americans have been physically victimized by the U.S. government and the military.) Third, they cite abuse of blacks by the American health profession, for example, the infamous Tuskegee Project. Tuskegee's influence extends far beyond the borders of the United States, reaching through Africa to Zimbabwe, where it is part of the maze of conspiracy theories. Though healthcare is supposed to be benevolent, conspiracy theories assume that medical personnel exist in two worlds, like actors who perform onstage but only reveal their real identity offstage. Worldwide, researchers report people suspect that healthcare representatives have some ulterior, presumably malign, purpose hidden behind their seemingly benevolent performance (Moscovici 1987:155–56; Pipes 1996:176, 201; Whetten-Goldstein and Nguyen 2002:172). AIDS conspiracy theories frequently suggest either direct subversive action, or non-action, in medical practice.

Letters to the editor inform readers that the real mastermind of the AIDS epidemic is the American government, exerting its control through far-reaching means such as the military. The news is not new. Readers hear about the request made by the U.S. Army, during a hearing of the House of Representatives' subcommittee on Department of Defense appropriations, June 9, 1969. The army asked for funding to develop a biological weapon that could target the human immune system.

Around the world, people assume that the army received the funds and developed the weapon: HIV/AIDS. Conspiracy theory thus traces the origin of the epidemic to June 1969 (Knight 2000:200–01). People perceive this as an attempt by the American government to eradicate humans of African descent around the world. Pseudoscientific publications available in Zimbabwe, such as Wolff Geisler's *AIDS: Origin, Spread and Healing* (1994), continue to disseminate this conspiracy theory with the support of the local press (Anonymous 1994a; Chiweza 1997:89).

Other reports in the Zimbabwean media refer to Fort Detrick, a U.S. military research laboratory in Maryland. People believe that researchers there have long investigated plagues and other forms of biological warfare (Anonymous 1986, 1987a). I spoke with two Zimbabweans who singled out this research center for its evil work; the information has spread far and wide. Believers think that the virus was either released accidentally or deliberately as part of a biological warfare program.[20] As far back as 1987, an American virologist working in Zimbabwe was trying to dismiss such claims as poor science, based on incorrect assumptions (*The Sunday Mail*, September 7, 1987).

Nonfiction, in the form of novels, also influences local perceptions about the epidemic. Novels that construct the whole history of AIDS as authored, intentional, and conspiratorial, are a source of popular conspiracy theories (Kruger 1996:248–49). Novels set in southern Africa, depicting an international collaboration of forces plotting to get rid of blacks, are available in Zimbabwe—for instance, Ben Geer's 1998 thriller *Something More Sinister*. Geer's novel argues that HIV/AIDS is a racist conspiracy targeting blacks. Nazi scientists and South African Boers used the knowledge of innocent and naïve scientists to fabricate a deadly virus affecting blacks. They then provided white Rhodesians with their products as a tool for fighting guerillas in their country, to limit the growth of the black Zimbabwean population, and to remain in power. This explains why non-black groups are suffering from HIV/AIDS; the lack of racial segregation allowed the virus to cross the race boundary. The novel further argues that HIV is just a single attempt to reach that goal within a wide array of more or less successful assaults: Ebola and other potential viruses serve the same purpose, which is another issue that respondents mentioned from time to time in interviews. This book was reviewed in local newspapers (Anonymous 1998). Some of my interviews show that people believe this novel's arguments. Other studies indicate that people elsewhere also believe the fiction (e.g., Karim 1993).

Such views are enmeshed in political propaganda. AIDS conspiracy fears have, as mentioned earlier, a strong connection to statements uttered by local and regional politicians. The Zimbabwean print media, in general, place greater emphasis in their HIV/AIDS reports on quoting government officials than on citing other, perhaps more authoritative, medical sources (Chari 2001:16). Therefore, Zimbabweans are frequently exposed to politicians' views about the AIDS epidemic. However, informants tend to remain somewhat skeptical about what politicians tell them. They said that information disseminated by politicians may be based less on factual evidence than on how well this information fits their political agenda; for example, the fact that Zimbabwean politicians politicize HIV/AIDS, attributing its origin to a Western plot, caused some informants to be critical of such views at best and reluctant to talk about them at worst. Here is a reaction typical of my informants:

> I don't really know where AIDS comes from, but I have heard that it originates in English-speaking countries, perhaps America. I am not sure who is behind it. I am not interested in politics and I do not want to know about it.

Residents develop distrust of what they read. They realize that politicians use HIV/AIDS, like many other issues, for their own purposes. Politicians do not agree about the causes of the epidemic or the actions to take. While government officials frequently refer to HIV/AIDS as a genocide attempt by a Western nation, the opposition party at times charges the Zimbabwean government itself with responsibility for the epidemic, mainly citing corruption and neglect. An example of the latter is the election poster of the MDC on page 121, the major opposition party. Some informants assume that the government may be implicated in an insidious plot involving HIV/AIDS. I noticed this among those who experienced the tortures and murders committed by the Fifth Brigade in southern Zimbabwe. Politically motivated violence during my fieldwork resulted in perceptions that the government could be responsible for HIV/AIDS:

> Some say the [Zimbabwean] government causes these diseases. They want to kill the people. Some say it started from Harare. I say "government" because they plotted to engineer viruses that led to AIDS.

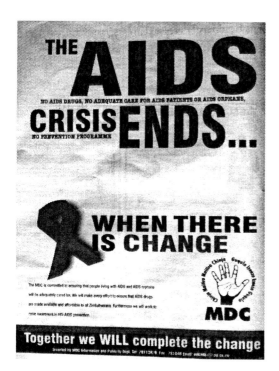

Opposition party's election campaign poster reflects the politicization of AIDS. *(Harare Daily News,* January 31, 2002)

These and other informants believe the government may again attempt genocide. Instead of the Fifth Brigade, the government is using HIV, which it had produced. The historical experience of Zimbabweans presents the familiar setting within which the epidemic gets anchored.

More commonly, the local imagination feeds on statements of government officials pointing at suspected conspiracies. The late vice-president of Zimbabwe, Mqabuko Joshua Nkomo, is a typical example of a Zimbabwean politician suspecting a conspiracy behind the AIDS epidemic; he stated explicitly that the prime motivation of the white conspirators was to wipe out the black population in Zimbabwe and to take its land and wealth (Anonymous 1996a; 1996c). Nkomo also expressed his conviction that whites have a treatment for HIV/AIDS but refuse to use it for individuals outside their own race. The latter argument directs us to a distinction between conspiracy theories: some argue that some evil human agency plans a malevolent act in a purposeful attempt to undermine a group, and others argue that evil agency deliberately refrains from acting to halt a malevolent event. Thus we have theories of "malicious intent," in contrast with theories of "benign neglect" (Turner 1993:189–90). Nkomo expressed his conviction that both types of conspiracies are happening, as did many people with whom I talked.

Similar utterances come from African politicians across the continent. Local Zimbabwean media featured conspiracy theories mentioned by the outspoken Libyan president Muammar Gaddafi, who accused the CIA of scientific experiments as part of their bacterial defense program; the scientists created HIV/AIDS as a means of spreading harm throughout the world (Anonymous 1990b; 2001a). His tendency to blame outsiders for HIV/AIDS became apparent when a Libyan court sentenced five Bulgarian nurses and a Palestinian doctor to death on charges they intentionally infected more than 400 children with the AIDS virus (Anonymous 2004). Former Namibian president Sam Nujoma was very vocal in asserting a Western conspiracy behind the epidemic (Anonymous 2001b). These statements by politicians have one idea in common; they suspect whites, particularly Americans, of deliberately infecting blacks as a part of a biological warfare program for their own gain. These statements are broadcast all over the continent.

Why is the United States suspected of being the mastermind behind the AIDS epidemic? The notion that AIDS is an American invention is a recurrent element in the international AIDS story (Farmer 1992:230; Kroeger 2003: 244; Treichler 1989:43). Why aren't former colonial regimes and their successors suspected of such plots? Vice President Nkomo gave this theory a specifically Zimbabwean flavor by arguing that the goal of spreading HIV/AIDS is to eradicate blacks and take their land and wealth. Whites took their land before, but that was a British act. Biological warfare is widely believed to have been used by the Rhodesian and South African whites during their struggle for majority rule in Zimbabwe and South Africa, respectively (Niehaus and Jonssen 2005:196–98; White 2004). It would only be a short step to conclude that whites now use HIV as their weapon to regain the land. So, why are the Americans largely thought to be involved in a conspiracy?

I believe that the popularity of attributing blame to Americans has first to do with the background of the many southern African politicians who were involved in the struggle to achieve majority rule. Most joined groups that were financially supported by the former Soviet Union and its allies during the Cold War. Many of them received military and academic training from communist nations hostile to America and the West. One of my assistants had joined a Zimbabwean guerilla force and then went to Moscow to obtain a degree in mass mobilization. I met others who trained in Eastern Europe, where they were exposed to anti-American propaganda, including certain conspiracy theories disseminated by the Soviet government among their allies. Upon their return to Africa, Zimbabweans shared these views with others. In the early years of the epidemic, the former Soviet Union circulated a story in twenty-five languages across eighty nations arguing that HIV was a biological warfare agent developed by the Central Intelligence Agency and the Pentagon (Chirimuuta and Chirimuuta 1989:8; Medvedev 1986). A study conducted in five Eastern European countries concluded that the belief that AIDS is a tool of biological warfare can be traced back to this prominent feature of the early Soviet reporting of HIV/AIDS (Goodwin et al. 2003). Such a conclusion makes sense in Zimbabwe.

Peoples' ideological bias against the United States may even be increasing because of another issue. It is easy to believe that Americans are malevolent because of the high prices for ARV drugs produced by American pharmaceutical companies. These companies appear to be unwilling to lower the costs for such drugs or to allow their generic production. Local Zimbabwean newspapers publish articles informing readers of attempts of Western firms to maintain their high prices for AIDS medications (Anonymous 1999d). It is assumed that these companies are protected by the U.S. government. Nkomo spoke about ARV drugs at the funeral of his son. He declared that the whites have a cure for AIDS but do not want to share it with the other races (Anonymous 1996a; 1996c). Such suspicions are expressed all over Africa and beyond.[21] Nkomo's view appears related to the high prices of American-produced ARV drugs, which most Africans cannot pay. The same view was reiterated by my informants, who expressed dismay and disgust that U.S. companies sell ARV drugs at high prices, making them unaffordable to most Zimbabweans. As Americans successfully withhold such drugs, people conclude that they also withhold a cure for AIDS. A painful thought for someone like Nkomo, whose son died of AIDS! Though his son most likely had easy access to antiretroviral drugs, Nkomo obviously became painfully aware of the struggle many Zimbabweans face as he dealt with the illness of his own son.

A contributing factor to blaming Americans for the AIDS epidemic is the barrage of political propaganda warning Zimbabweans of ongoing racial discrimination against them, by whites in general and Americans and Britons in particular. Zimbabweans understand discrimination because their history of racial segregation and exclusion from public decision-making only ended in 1980 when majority rule was achieved in Zimbabwe. Injustices committed by the former white regime are very much alive in the memory of the older generation, who share their sentiments with younger associates. It is only a short step to conclude that nations who hate blacks are plotting to eradicate all Africans.

Why do local politicians get involved with conspiracy theories? Scholars argue that this happens when a government suspects external and internal forces are plotting against it (Jaworski 2001:23; Mason 2002:42). The same has been argued for cases when sorcery suspicions are fostered by a society's leadership (Harris 1975:240). The current Zimbabwean government has lost support among the electorate, pursues a policy of surveillance and intimidation against its citizens, and has a paranoid fear that Western governments plan to topple it. Such a government is predisposed to disseminating conspiracy theories. The propagation of conspiracy theories by those in power may itself be evidence of a larger conspiracy, namely, they may represent a tactic by politicians to divert public opinion from the government and unite the nation by creating a common enemy.[22] In other words, the Zimbabwean government exploited racial and ethnic issues as well as historic injustices in order to blame outsiders for national problems. The aim was to rally support among the electorate.

Political convictions determine to some degree whether an informant admitted believing that HIV/AIDS is the result of a conspiracy. I noticed that interviewees, such as war veterans, who approved government policies showed stronger belief in conspiracy theories involving foreigners than did the community as a whole. Their suspicion of biological warfare during the liberation struggle (White 2004) makes such views more credible to them. In addition, their closeness to the governing party and its representatives is reflected in their acceptance of statements made by politicians. The war veterans seem to have a stronger tendency than the general population to draw from media sources close to the government, particularly from daily newspapers such as *The Chronicle*. A more critical view of the AIDS conspiracies promoted by the government is presented in media favoring the political opposition, such as *The Daily News*. However, many war veterans frown on the opposition media. After all, as one of them said with a smile on his face, "*The Daily News* is the mouthpiece of 'the enemy'!"

Nkulumane theories, like AIDS conspiracy suspicions elsewhere, are diverse, variegated, and contradictory, making it difficult to present them in a systematic manner. However, there is a common denominator among most people in Nkulumane who believe in theories about the origin of HIV; they generally believe that the virus originated outside the country. Residents often said that HIV *kwavela emazweni* (came from other nations), or *kwavela ephetsheya* (came from beyond). Exactly where outside the country HIV came from was not commonly agreed upon. Two generalized arguments surfaced.

Some argued that HIV/AIDS originated in African countries. If respondents referred to neighboring countries such as Botswana, South Africa, and to a lesser degree Zambia, Mozambique and Namibia, they usually observed that many Zimbabwean migrant laborers return from these countries sick with AIDS. Nkulumane residents, seeing many of these migrant laborers terminally ill, logically concluded that HIV must have entered Zimbabwe via its neighbors. Similarly, they pointed to the Democratic Republic of Congo (DRC), not a direct but a regional neighbor, as an immediate entry point for the epidemic. Zimbabwean soldiers were involved in the military confrontation in the DRC from 1998 to 2002 (MacLean 2002:522–24); many returned showing symptoms of AIDS-related diseases. The general feeling in the township was that soldiers have a higher incidence of AIDS than men in the general population. Several times I was told that residential areas with a high proportion of soldiers have a high proportion of widows, many of whom lost their husbands not to war but to AIDS.

Others posited that HIV came from *beyond*, a term that commonly carries a specific meaning, namely, overseas nations. These are, in Ndebele, the nations that are *phetsheya kolwandle* (beyond the ocean). Initially in an interview I was not always sure what residents referred to, neighboring countries or overseas nations, but this would become apparent in the course of conversation. When people referred to African countries, they usually said these were places where HIV is prevalent, so they thought Zimbabwean soldiers acquired the disease there, primarily by sexual transmission. When they referred to overseas countries, they generally pointed to them as areas where they thought HIV originated, where it was purposely engineered and administered.

Researchers have observed a similar distinction elsewhere in discussions of AIDS beliefs. Blame for the epidemic is attributed to some sort of "other," so typical in sorcery and conspiracy beliefs, to a distant "other" for manufacturing HIV, and to a close "other" as the avenue through which the virus enters an individual's life.

Some interviewees related the origin of the epidemic to an accident that either led to the creation of HIV or resulted in the unintentional escape of the virus from a laboratory. Such reports are not unique to Zimbabwe but come from other African countries as well.[23]

Such theories are based upon the knowledge that Western scientists use animals in experiments to find cures or test new medicines. Zimbabweans have heard discussions about HIV being related to animal—mainly primate—viruses that could have crossed to humans in experiments. An informant told me a common Zimbabwean variant of the "accident theory":

> The white is very smart! Especially the American is very clever and
> well-educated. When he wants to find out about the nature of something, he tests it first on animals. When the animal survives the test
> without harm, the same thing is tried on humans. It is given to humans either through ingesting blood of this animal or through other

ways, to see its effect on humans—how much time it takes to see some reactions, and what symptoms the humans develop indicating that they are now infected.

This and comparable interview quotes argue that medical scientists did experiments using animals, apparently with good intentions. If the experiment was successful, then a subsequent experiment was conducted involving humans. Scientists erred during the second experiment, so humans became infected. A closer look and a comparison with other quotes show that various hidden lines of thought can be identified in the quote.

First, the whites are thought to be clever. Although the term is generally a positive one, covering a whole gamut of meaning from being gifted and educated to being wise, it sometimes carries a negative meaning. In this sense, if someone is called "clever" the speaker means that the person is using knowledge and experience for selfish purposes. This metaphorical use of the term points at the danger of knowledge used egoistically or even maliciously against others. A sociocentric society that is consensus-based, emphasizing the common welfare of its members, is aware of the potential abuse of knowledge and expertise.

The current economic conditions, which necessitate cooperation with other members in order to make ends meet, feed into such views. There is ample evidence of the abuse of knowledge, education, and power in the past by a "clever" racial minority and in the present by the "clever" political and economic elite. They appear to be cleverly enriching themselves without considering the common well-being. In many statements on the origin of HIV/AIDS, the whites were thought to be "clever" and instrumental in its genesis, implying that they did not consider the welfare of others but were concerned just about their own benefits.

Through further questioning I elicited what type or group of whites are more likely to be involved in these "clever" experiments. The ones closest at home are Zimbabwean whites, yet they were not thought to be responsible for unleashing HIV; the culprits are Westerners, particularly Americans. Blame falls mainly on the technologically advanced Western nations that conduct the medical experiments reported in the newspapers:

> Baboons clinically infected with the AIDS virus became the first ani-
> mals to develop full-blown symptoms of the disease, prompting hopes
> of a quick testing of new drugs and vaccines, researchers said yester-
> day. (Anonymous 1994b)

Conspiracy theories commonly identify parallels between unrelated or loosely related events. Thus, news reports involving monkeys and primates in AIDS experiments get attached to other information, particularly to one scientific theory locating the origin of HIV in simian retroviruses, especially the African green monkey. This theory has met strong criticism among African scholars, who demonstrate flaws and hidden racism in it.[24] Zimbabwean media reports critically dismissed this theory as racist (Anonymous 1986) and refuted other theories that locate the origin of HIV/AIDS in Africa for similar reasons. Consider the following excerpt from a news report in the early years of the epidemic:

> What filth are our former colonial masters, and present neo-colonial
> exploiters, trying to pin on Africa? The collusion of the major Western
> capitalist states with Apartheid South Africa has been magnificently ex-
> posed by Cde. Mugabe, Cde. Kaunda and other African patriots, as well
> as the African National Congress of South Africa. (Anonymous 1986:35)

When people spoke about AIDS experiments with primates, they quickly connected this information with the accusation that HIV originated somewhere in Africa. The depiction of Africa as the cradle of AIDS and the resulting anti-African prejudice caused many Africans to express their indignation. Many insisted that the virus was sent to Africa from the West, a counterattack against what they felt were accusatory and demeaning statements by white Westerners.[25]

Who is better equipped than educated individuals in the West to do such experiments? The reason for the experiments and the mystery surrounding them was explained to me by a focus group of middle-aged women:

> These countries do like to experiment. I am not sure what they were
> experimenting, only that they experimented with animals. Then they

took the disease from animals and injected it into humans. From these humans it then spread to others.

Suspicions about the Western scientists were boosted by reports that medical research accidentally led to an outbreak of AIDS in central Africa (Bennet 2003:282; Wright 1987). Similarly, promising reports on the prospects of biologically engineering viruses in the local newspaper added credibility to AIDS conspiracy theories touted in the mass media. People read that such experiments can lead to the creation of a more dangerous form of HIV (Kimbrell 1993). Some residents, like the interviewee above, assumed a general curiosity of Westerners to discover hidden knowledge, to be interested in testing new thoughts and practices, and to strive for progress and development—albeit for their own selfish goals. This is the context within which HIV/AIDS was first discovered, they believe, and then accidentally entered humanity.

After the experiments on animals were carried out, the next step of the "clever" whites, according to prevailing conspiracy theories, was to test the knowledge gained through animal experiments on human guinea pigs. Similar beliefs about the etiology of the human AIDS epidemic are reported from other parts of the world (e.g., Wilson and Hill 1998:105). People told me that, when humans were infected with the virus, it spread easily from one person to another; the AIDS epidemic began to take its course.

These arguments imply that if Westerners had not searched for knowledge through testing, but adhered to proven and inherited beliefs and customs, all this would not have happened. The "clever" (meaning selfish) search for the new and unknown is risky and dangerous for society, and HIV/AIDS is the best example for a bad outcome.

Interpreting such theories as metaphors about the consequences of behavior that ignores inherited values, beliefs, and practices—that is, searching for the unknown—is also seen in other accounts that carry additional meanings. Consider the following, from an interview with a focus group of mixed youth:

AIDS started with scientists who did medical experiments using monkeys, trying to find out more about this disease. However, later AIDS shifted from these monkeys to human beings. Most probably because of those who enjoy "playing a bit" with animals, like veterinary doctors, the virus crossed over to humans.

The youth mentioned the following sequence of events: medical experiments with primates were followed by veterinary doctors "playing" with the primates, resulting in the transmission of HIV from primates to humans. According to informants holding such beliefs, the scientists were aware of the virus and tested it on primates. They did not deliberately infect humans with the virus, but it crossed over from primates to humans because both species were somehow in close proximity to each other.

In a normal setting, this is thought to be impossible; humans live in civilized villages and cities while monkeys and primates live in the uncivilized veldt. Only rarely do the two species meet because their habitats are so different. Only when we ignore or even abandon our values, beliefs, and practices, and change the human habitat into a wilderness and human society into a band of baboons, do the boundaries break down. A humorous example of such a view is the following excerpt from a newspaper article:

> A chief in parliament yesterday speculated that the baboon seen in Harare's Avenues on Monday morning was a manifestation of people in modern Zimbabwe [who are] breaking taboos, traditional values, and norms. . . . "What people are doing these days is what is bringing baboons into Harare," he said amid laughter. (Anonymous 1994d)

This traditional chief, a representative in the upper house of the parliament, used satire to underscore his message that Zimbabwe had become so decadent as to blur the distinction between human society and a baboon band! My respondents told me that the scientists, who were selfishly "clever" in abandoning traditional norms, transformed human society into a wild and lawless group, somehow bridging the gap between humans and primates. If the scientists had not bridged the gap, they thought, HIV/AIDS would never have crossed to humanity. The question arises if this metaphor of bridging the gap carries additional meanings.

Most interviewees used such statements to address a general loss of values. Some, however, had something tangible in mind. The Ndebele term for *playing* is, like its English equivalent, ambiguous and can express sexual connotations. Veterinarians are, by virtue of their profession, "playing" with animals in the sense of working on them. However, this statement could also be a covert reference to acts of bestiality as the origin of AIDS. Variants of this theory use other terms that also carry sexual connotations, such as *meeting* and *eating*. HIV/AIDS is a sexually transmitted disease and any sexual notion can get connected to the epidemic. To connect the origin of the epidemic to the belief that HIV has its origin in the animal kingdom is easy. In Chapter 9, I present a narrative that involves women being paid to sleep with dogs. Such beliefs are not unique to Zimbabwe and have been observed elsewhere in the world (e.g., Medina 2002:88, 109). In other words, Western scientists, Western veterinarians, and others who are in close contact with wild animals violated traditional values and caused the beginning of the human HIV/AIDS epidemic. These theories postulate that the virus already existed in the animal kingdom, emerged in the course of medical experiments with infected animals, and entered humans through bestiality. HIV then quickly spread from one person to another through heterosexual intercourse, as several respondents emphasized.

The accident theories in Nkulumane interviews relate the origin of HIV to violations of inherited values, beliefs, and practices. We are again reminded how strongly such interpretations of the AIDS epidemic resemble the sorcery paradigm. The scientists are characterized, like sorcerers, as selfish, greedy, and immoral. If Western scientists had not been so "clever," selfishly searching for new knowledge and expertise; if they had adhered to traditional values, beliefs, and practices; if they and others had not broken taboos; then HIV/AIDS would never have become a problem for humanity.

The breaking of taboos could refer to individuals not adhering to tradition, but it could also hint at deep-rooted developments in society. The accident theory may indicate fundamental changes in society; that is, it may be a metaphor for cultural change. Rapid culture change can trigger a crisis in the *Weltanschauung* of residents and in their value and belief systems, providing, according to some scholars, a fertile ground for formulating conspiracy theories. Seen as such, the Westerners and the educated professionals represent a threat to a traditional society and are thus blamed for the evils of society, including AIDS! While some informants appear to view such theories as metaphors, others took them literally, believing medical experiments to be the source of the human AIDS epidemic.

Notes

1. Psychological interpretations of conspiracy beliefs are discussed, e.g., by Abalakina-Paap et al 1999:639; Crocker et al 1999:950; Goertzel 1994; Graumann 1987:245; Jaworski 2001:13; Knight 2000:18; Kramer 1994:222; Robins and Post 1997:14–15; and Young 1990:156.

2. This line of interpretation has been applied to both sorcery and conspiracy suspicions in Crocker et al 1999:949; DeParle 1990:B7; Farmer 1992:247; Fernando 1993; Fry 1975; Guinan 1993; Hooper 1999; Knight 2000:148–53; Pipes 1996:325; Sasson 1995:265; Turner 1993; Waters 1997:112–21; and Zonis and Joseph 1994:453.

3. Scholars of both sorcery and conspiracies have argued this, e.g., Bogucka 2001:127–28; Bourdillon 1993:110; Crawford 1967:69; Evans-Pritchard 1951:100; Kluckhohn 1944:107; LeVine 1982:273; Malinowski 1969:188; Parish 2001:6; Parker 2001:199; and Zonis and Joseph 1994:447.

4. See, for example, Gluckman 1966; Hofstadter 1965:34–39; Mary Aquina 1968:47; Pipes 1996:303-304; Popper 1962:341 and 1966:94.

5. This argument has been brought forward for both types of causal explanation, e.g., by Gluckman 1966; Goertzel 1994:739; Graumann 1987:247; Groh 1987:1, 2001:193; Kluckhohn 1944:82–87; Mary Aquina 1968:47; Mayer 1970:50; Melley 2000:16–17; Moscovici 1987:151–52, 160–61; Robins and Post 1997:52, 301; and Sidky 1997:89.

6. See, e.g., Ashforth 2005: 275; Gluckman 1966; Hendershot 1999:21; Kluckhohn 1944:82; Mary Aquina 1968:47; and Marcus 1999:5.

7. This has been convincingly argued, e.g., by Goldstein 2004:36; Knopf 1975; Niehaus and Jonssen 2005:180–81; and Sasson 1995:265.

8. The quotes of the Ugandan and Kenneth Kaunda are both in Sabatier and Tinker 1988:148.

9. Key studies presenting this argument are, e.g., Beck 1985:186; du Toit 1971; Glick 1967:36; and Mitchell 1960:194.

10. Key studies are Altman 1986:43; Bogart and Thorburn 2003b:1063; Gadon et al. 2001:794; Goertzel 1994:732–34; Herek and Capitano 1994; Klonoff and Landrine 1999; Mays and Cochran 1996; Turner 1993:159; and Whetten-Goldstein and Nguyen 2002:173.

11. This argument has been brought forward, e.g., in Bogart and Thorburn 2003b:1061; Crocker et al. 1999; Farmer 1992:232; Gasch et al. 1991; Herek and Glunt 1991; Herek and Capitanio 1994; Klonoff and Landrine 1999a; Parsons et al. 1999; Sengupta et al. 2000:279; and Thomas and Quinn 1991.

12. Among key studies arguing this point are Abalakina-Paap and Stephan 1999; Jameson 1988:356; Jaworski 2001:22, 26; LeVine 1982:271; Mason 2002:50-51; Melley 2000:11–13; 2002:62-63; Parsons et al. 1999:217; and Zonis and Joseph 1994:430.

13. Scholars interpreting sorcery and conspiracy suspicions have observed this dynamics, see, e.g., Abalakina-Paap et al. 1999:644; Bratich 2002:134–40; Brunvand 1981; Butt 2005:414; Fine 1992; Goldstein 2004:36, 98; Groh 1987:3, 2001:189; Kapferer 1990; Kroeger 2003:243; Masquelier 2000; Parsons et al. 1999:218; Perice 1997; Taussig 1987; and White 2000:68, 85.

14. See Cantwell 1988, 1993, 2002:87; Cress-Welsing 1991:298–301; Gilbert 1996:55–56, 1998; and Porter 2001:22–23.

15. See, for example, Bogart and Thorburn 2005:216; Freimuth et al. 2001:799, 805; Gray 1998; Herek and Capitanio 1994; Jones 1981; Joffe 1999:50; Klonoff and Landrine 1999:451–56; Medina 2002:4; Thomas and Curran 1999; and Washington 1998:71–74.

16. This core argument is presented, e.g., in Bratich 2002:138–39; Buckley 1997; Butt 2005:412; Goldstein 2004:52, 92; Lindenbaum 1998, 2001; Setel 1999; Taussig 1992; and Treichler 1999:319.

17. Though also applicable to sorcery beliefs, this has been mainly argued for conspiracy theories. See, e.g., in Abalakina-Paap et al. 1999:646; Coleman 1976:20; Evans-Pritchard 1976b:150; Gluckman 1966:102–105; Goldberg 2001:240; Goertzel 1994:739–41; Graumann and Moscovici 1987:ix; Groh 1987:5; Melley 2000:8; Pipes 1996:251; and Skinnner 2001:106–108.

18. This has been argued, e.g., by AIDS Control and Prevention Project 1998:22; Meursing 1997:61–62; Nicoll et al. 1993:236; and Pitts and Jackson 1993a:213.

19. See, e.g., Chari 2001:14, 106; Gregson et al. 1998; Nangati 1991; Ndlovu and Sihlangu 1992; Pitts et al. 1991; and Pitts and Jackson 1993a.

20. Such views have been encouraged by, e.g., Anonymous 1987; Bennet 2003:279–81; Duesberg 1987, 1996:379; Segal 1990; and Strecker 1986; Scholars from various disciplines interpreted this understanding, e.g., Goldstein 2004:91; Vankin and Whalen 1995:299; and Wilson and Hill 1998:34.

21. This has been documented, e.g., by Dilger 1999a:7; Meursing 1997:340; Sabatier and Tinker 1988:63–66; and Whetten-Goldstein and Nguyen 2002:174.

22. See, e.g., Blackmore and Dawkins 1999:4–7; Graumann 198 7:249–50; Graumann and Moscovici 1987:viii; Lush 2001:493; and Pipes 1996:358–59.

23. See, for example, Grundlingh 1999:68; Medina 2002; and Mputu n.d.:3, 7.

24. This has, e.g., been argued by Noireau 1987. This and comparable theories have been summarized in Duh 1991:60–62. Examples of scholars dissenting with such arguments are Chirimuuta and Chirimuuta 1989:130; Engelhard et al. 1988; and Sabatier and Tinker 1988:52–54, 89.

25. Key studies containing this argument are Farmer 1992:247; Nations and Monte 1997:445; Schoepf 1995:37; and Sontag 1990:140.

CHAPTER 7

Conspiracy Theories Involving Healthcare Providers

Most of the origin beliefs expressed to me during my fieldwork in Zimbabwe were conspiracy theories. Some theories implicated medical workers, just as did those discussed in the literature (e.g., van den Borne 2005: 61–62; Wilson and Hill 1998:57, 245). Conspiracy suspicions pointing at healthcare providers have a long history, as I found out while reading in the National Archives in Harare. I was surprised to learn that present-day responses to HIV/AIDS were similar to those of Zimbabweans during the epidemic of Spanish influenza in 1918–1919. Across the country, individuals desperately ill with flu had refused the healthcare provided by British colonizers. The native Zimbabweans believed that the medicines were poisonous, and administered with the intent to kill. It was generally said that it was sure death to take such drugs.[1] A certain Reverend Skold reported nearly a century ago:

> One day I found quite a number of natives ploughing in a garden, but at the sight of my cart they all ran away, except an old woman. When I asked her why they ran away, she replied to me "We have heard that *Umfundisi*[2] was coming with medicine but we do not want the white men's medicine which only kills us." (Skold 1918)

Suspicion of the early colonizers—who subjugated the ethnic groups they encountered, appropriated their land, and relegated them to subordinate and inferior positions—is understandable. Their arrival brought great loss to the indigenous people; naturally, anything provided by the intruders could be seen as potentially harmful. Accounts related to HIV/AIDS show the same pattern: negative experiences with dominant outsiders resulted in mistrust and suspicion. The fact that many medical doctors currently in Zimbabwe are of European[3] descent feeds into perceptions that health professionals purposely further the spread of the epidemic. Statements about this from people of diverse backgrounds featured prominently in my interviews:

> We black people know how to bewitch each other, but white people also know how to use sorcery, especially the doctors. When a doctor wants to kill me these days, he just gives me an injection and I die. So, there is someone who is very mean and "smart," who is really "clever," like the doctors. He knows where to get the viruses.

> It happens that someone gets the wrong treatment in the hospital. He may be given an injection, which is not what he needs for his illness. This is not an accident; I have heard that you get a lot of money when you do so. So, people are aware that you get a lot of money when you kill someone. The undertakers pay you. They tell you to kill someone and then you will be given a lot of money.

The first quote implicitly connects "white people" to harmful practices such as sorcery. It is another example of conspiracy theories closely related to sorcery beliefs. In this case, both the conspirator and the sorcerer are secretly plotting to kill their unwitting victims in order to benefit from their deaths. Thus the genesis of some conspiracy theories lies in distrust of the medical profession.

Zimbabweans know that medical workers have access to the HIV virus; they have the capacity to inject infected blood into unaware patients, who may even be unconscious. Like sorcerers, the medical specialists are "smart or "clever" in the pejorative sense described earlier. This attribution of smartness implies the selfishness of medical researchers, who benefit through their expertise. Race is not an issue; physicians of any ancestry may be perceived like traditional sorcerers because they appear to reap rewards for themselves by inflicting harm on unassuming victims.

Yet other factors have contributed to the perception that healthcare workers have a vested interest in the spread of HIV/AIDS. Popular mistrust of the medical profession in Zimbabwe was exacerbated by several scandals of medical professionals doing experiments without their patients' consent. The local media covered such cases extensively through the years, as in the following newspaper report:

> Thirteen terminally-ill patients, ten of them HIV-positive, died after a doctor allegedly experimented on them with injections of an unusual drug, *povidone iodine*.[4] (Nkala 1999)

The most prominent case was of a medical doctor with doubtful credentials, a physician named McGown, who worked during the 1980s and 1990s in various Zimbabwean hospitals and clinics, doing morphine experiments on more than 500 unsuspecting patients (Mutizwa-Mangiza 1999:134–36). Coincidentally, this was the period when HIV/AIDS became known in Zimbabwe, which allowed people to create a cognitive link between the two events. McGown made headlines over an extended period of time,[5] and people still mentioned him during my interviews in 2003.

The legacy of McGown and other "smart" medical professionals is mistrust of the healthcare system, which motivated the development of some AIDS conspiracy theories. Local examples of abuses by medical professionals explain the ease with which reports of medical experiments elsewhere (for example, the Tuskegee project) were believed by Zimbabweans. Credibility of the reports grew because accusations of covert healthcare discrimination against non-white minority groups, published in the local papers (e.g., Anonymous 1999a), fed into allegations of a conspiracy.

At times, the argument shifts from shady experiments to other ways of being "smart." Recall that some Nkulumane residents argued healthcare providers make money by injecting people with HIV. Again, parallels with the sorcery paradigm are evident—particularly the assumed selfishness and greed of sorcerers. It is said that conspirators are like sorcerers, illicitly accumulating wealth (Moore and Sanders 2001:11–18). They are being paid by those who have a vested interest in infecting people, that is, the undertakers who profit financially from the human suffering of HIV/AIDS. Media reports that some sectors of society thrive because of HIV/AIDS nurture this attitude:

> Coffin manufacturers are opening corner shops in high-density suburbs in the urban areas to cash in on the booming business. "Undertaking is now one of the most competitive markets," says Victor Chitongo of the Chitkem group of security companies, who is still setting up his funeral undertaking business. (Munthali 1996)

Residents are ruefully aware that HIV/AIDS means big business for some sectors of society, especially those associated with funeral practices. Cemeteries fill up quickly in Bulawayo, as in the other cities of Zimbabwe (Anonymous 1999b), and undertaker firms are flourishing. A brief drive I had planned into Luveve cemetery, burial ground for low-income Bulawayo residents, turned into a lengthy tour visiting graves. Far from the solemnity of funerals, a lively hustle and bustle characterized activities at the cemetery.

Frequently, several funerals are being conducted simultaneously. Although the funeral parties appear to be respectful of each other, the singing of religious hymns, the search for shovels and soil to fill the grave, the preaching and eulogies, as well as the relentless comings and goings, are irritating. Several people bemoaned to me the lack of respect traditionally shown at funerals, saying that the loss of a loved one has become, for some, an opportunity to raise funds, a practice unthinkable some years ago.

In addition to the money made by those who conduct funeral services, other cemetery entrepreneurs find a niche for generating income; for instance, small-scale vendors plant vegetables alongside graves and sell packaged food and drink (Dongozi 2003). Even though the harsh economic climate in Zimbabwe has forced people to use their ingenuity for raising money, Nkulumane residents frequently criticized those who seemed to have no scruples about how they did it.

This criticism applies to individual vendors, but it is also directed at established businesses, such as undertakers and carpenters. Some of them become wealthy. I was walking through an affluent suburb of Bulawayo with a companion who showed me an extravagant mansion being built by the owner of an undertaking firm. These firms appear to "make a killing at the cemetery," to cite the title of a newspaper article bemoaning such developments (Dongozi 2003). It is not surprising, then, that some informants concluded those who profit from the epidemic may be implicated in the genesis of HIV/AIDS. They suspect healthcare providers of collaborating in order to get their share of the profits made through AIDS deaths.

Some people argue that healthcare providers directly increase their profits through the AIDS epidemic. These profiteers are happy that prices for healthcare, especially the drugs, are skyrocketing; medical personnel thrive because of HIV/AIDS. In contrast, regular citizens are worse off financially because of the current economic crisis in the country. Some interviewees concluded that healthcare providers must have some complicity with the AIDS epidemic because they appear to "make a killing" through HIV/AIDS.

The costs for healthcare have soared because of the desperate state of the Zimbabwean healthcare system. While a few can afford the relatively expensive private healthcare, the average person relies on government hospitals that are understaffed, overcrowded, and lacking even the most basic amenities. One nurse in a government hospital told me that the state of healthcare there is "deplorable," and several patients have died because of it. Such conditions lower the morale of those working in the public healthcare system, which in turn negatively affects patient care.

People suspicious of medical personnel blame them for this dreadful situation: some accuse them of not caring for patients, privately selling medicine, or wrongly administering drugs. It is not surprising that some township residents make a connection between the appalling conditions and HIV/AIDS and want to attribute some responsibility for the spread of HIV to medical personnel. Taken together with other factors, this encourages suspicions that healthcare providers must have a vested interest in furthering the spread of HIV/AIDS. Such suspicions are, however, less numerous and less overt than conspiracy beliefs that attribute active responsibility to outside forces in the spread of the epidemic.

Notes

1. While researching documents in the National Archives in Harare, I found several examples of such perceptions, e.g., Campbell 1918; Loveless 1918; and Scogings 1918.

2. *Umfundisi* refers to any minister of religion. The term is derived from the Ndebele verb *ukufundisa*, meaning "to teach."

3. Actually, a substantial number of medical doctors are of other non-black descent. However, in the local perception, particularly in rural areas, the term *European* can even include people of Middle Eastern, Indian, and other relatively light-skinned groups.

4. *Povidone iodine* is an antiseptic used to treat bacterial and chlamydeous conjunctivitis, especially in underdeveloped countries where antibiotics are often unavailable or too costly.

5. See, e.g., Anonymous 1994c and 1997a.

CHAPTER 8

Conspiracy Theories Involving Westerners

Most residents' theories explaining the genesis of HIV/AIDS in Nkulumane were neither accident theories nor theories implicating health professionals. Instead, these theories linked the epidemic to other culprits, most of whom were from Western, developed nations. Frequently, Zimbabweans suspected white people—usually Americans—and their governments of evil acts that somehow triggered the epidemic. These agents were considered "smart," with the pejorative connotation explained earlier and its resonance with sorcery beliefs. People with whom I spoke thought these agents had a vested interest in harming black Zimbabweans. Similar views have been reported elsewhere and are not specific to Zimbabwe.[1]

Such beliefs are not entirely the product of fantasy, being at least partly grounded in the objective reality of the believers' history, particularly regarding the selection of groups depicted as villains. We have seen that social groups adhere to conspiracy models partly because of a history of oppression and partly because of their anguishing daily experience. During my discussions in Nkulumane, people spoke of a long history of racially motivated alienation and segregation. Majority rule was achieved only in 1980, and memories of their colonial history are very much alive. Many elderly people still remembered when they were forcibly removed from their rural homes during the establishment of white-owned commercial farms. War veterans who actively took part in the struggle for majority rule remember the atrocities committed by the white minority regime during the guerilla war. They dedicated years of their lives to fight a regime that had placed blacks at the margins of society. Various residents in the township experienced racism and discrimination in the workplace even after majority rule was achieved. Until a few years ago, whites remained the economic elite, and some of them looked down on other races. Their occasional derogatory statements about other races spread quickly through word of mouth.

Although the youth and children did not personally experience what their parents, grandparents, relatives, and in-laws had, they still heard about incidents of racism. They hear stories from their elders, learn about historic events in school, and are exposed to stories in the media—which frequently report stories about racism and discrimination, from historic and current times, from Zimbabwe and overseas. Residents are very much aware of racism and discrimination against blacks in other parts of the world, particularly in America. Thus, it is not surprising that both young and old conclude that accusations blaming whites for HIV/AIDS are credible. Or, as one interviewee said, "We black people were not treated well by the whites; something evil like giving us AIDS does not bother whites."

It is striking to note in the interview texts that racist notions are expressed in ontological terms: one informant told me whites despise blacks and regard them as a "curse for humanity." I heard that whites place blacks on the same level as animals; therefore, harming blacks is like "mistreating an animal," said one informant. I heard Zimbabweans recall hearing white Zimbabweans call blacks "baboons." Although I personally never heard such a derogatory statement from white Zimbabweans, historical evidence of such sentiments exists (Kaler 1998:354; Ranger 1999:95).

In southern Zimbabweans' thinking the boundary between baboons and humans is not as clear-cut as in Western thinking; there is some evidence among the Shona that baboon spirits have been approached in appeasement and propitiation ceremonies (Bullock 1950:160; Maingard

1929:840). Local tales and traditional knowledge teach that baboons are distant cousins of humans who live in the wilderness in chaotic bands without norms and values, in contrast to human society, which follows inherited norms and values (Ndhlukula 1980:18–19). It, nevertheless, remains an insult if a white person calls a black "baboon." People are fully aware of what is implied. Black Zimbabweans assume they have an answer to why whites, their fellow human beings, have mistreated them. Whites see blacks, not as their fellows, but as beings on a lower level. This explains historic and present injustices, because, as blacks say, "Maltreating us did not give them a bad conscience. It is like treating animals."

The distance between whites and blacks is also evident in the interviewees' choice of words to address them. While in Ndebele *abantu* is widely used as a generic word for all black Africans, generally whites are not included. However, at times one hears *abantu abamhlophe* (white people) in contrast to *abantu abansundu* (brown people), or *abantu abamnyama* (black people). Whites are, however, generally not a part of the *abantu* category and mostly addressed as *abelungu,* or less respectfully as *amakhiwa.*

Abelungu referred originally to a puppy, most likely due to the whites' inability to function maturely in an indigenous society, much like a little puppy clumsily relates with other dogs. *Amakhiwa* is related to the fruit of the fig tree, probably because of the color of its fruit, which bears some resemblance to the skin color of Europeans. The general tendency is for black Zimbabweans to express a difference linguistically between whites and black Africans.

A similar tendency occurs in the Shona language as well as in other southern African vernaculars (e.g., Comaroff and Comaroff 1992:53). The persistence of such linguistic distinctions indicates that more than twenty years after majority rule, people with whom I spoke still see a gap between whites and blacks. This gap contributes to the tendency of Zimbabwean blacks to assign causal responsibility for the AIDS epidemic to whites.

Some people told me that whites have a specific reason to exclude and discriminate against blacks. The whites did so out of greed: greed for land, greed for power, greed for money. They accumulated much wealth by taking it away from others and were reluctant to share it. In other words, they are "smart" in the pejorative sense. Greed is often assumed to be the motivation behind sorcery; thus, a possible conclusion is that those who are greedy are sorcerers. For instance, an elderly man compared whites in general to greedy sorcerers:

> AIDS comes from people, especially the whites, who prepare "chemicals." They are like sorcerers who want to get rid of others. For example, I am a sorcerer if I want to get rid of you. The sorcerers are full of jealousy and have a bad spirit.

The greedy sorcerer wants to obtain the object of its greed and desire by "getting rid of," or sacrificing, the person to whom it rightfully belongs. Whites have produced "chemicals" to eliminate black Zimbabweans. The term *chemical* enables another connection to sorcery. In the vernacular of Ndebele, *chemical* is expressed by using either the English adaptation *ikhemikhal* or the generic term for any medicinal substance, *umuthi*. "Medicine" can be used for both negative and positive goals. The last quote clearly refers to a negative use, a poison that was produced and used to cause harm and to take the victims' valuables. The resemblance of this and related accounts to sorcery arguments is evident.

Many people with whom I talked suspected that the central target of outsider greed is land. The culprits push the spread of AIDS in order to get Zimbabwe's land, coveting its agricultural areas, mineral resources, and other assets. In the propaganda of the ruling ZANU-PF party in Zimbabwe, land is frequently mentioned as the wealth of black Zimbabweans that is the object of others' envy. This propaganda is ever-present in government-directed radio and TV broadcasts as well as print. People listening to the radio or watching the local TV station hear hours of government propaganda about the imperative of black ownership of land.

This political propaganda bedevils the small white farming community and, implicitly, the former colonial power, Great Britain. People believe these white farmers are engaged in a plot to retake Zimbabwe, its land, and its government. Government propaganda further encourages the view that HIV/AIDS is a deliberate plot. Whites want to prevent further loss of their power. The tragic coincidence of the first appearance of HIV/AIDS with the struggle for achieving majority rule created a cruel connection in some minds:

> AIDS wasn't here some time ago. AIDS was discovered in the 1970s. This was the time of the liberation war, and because of biological warfare, maybe scientists wanted to use it as a weapon to fight against insurgences and guerrilla movements here and there.

> I am a Freedom Fighter[2] and I believe that AIDS is something which was deliberately "planted" during the war. It was "sown" by our enemy; his aim was kill us, to finish us.

Such arguments echo the AIDS conspiracy presented in the novel mentioned in Chapter 6 (Geer 1998). The novel refers to the last years of the white regime in Rhodesia, when its rule was increasingly under pressure. The author argues that, to counter the opposition forces, the Rhodesian army resolved to use biological warfare. The novel may not be far off what actually happened. When it became evident during the war that the white government was unable to hold onto power, some sections of the Rhodesian army appear to have secretly resolved to use biological warfare as a last resort (White 2004:230–31). It is not surprising that suspicions of biological warfare lend further credence to local ideas about human agency in the origins and distributions of HIV/AIDS.

The battle was nevertheless lost and majority rule achieved. Some people with whom I discussed it took this historic struggle into account:

> When we got independence we achieved majority rule and could select our own government. Some whites did not want this. And you see who is dying today in Africa—only blacks are dying, not the whites! They are happy that we are dying so that they become the majority and rule our country again.

Zimbabweans concluded that some whites did not appreciate being subject to the new government and used HIV to reverse the situation by eliminating either the new black leaders or the whole black population. As HIV continues to kill mostly blacks, the Rhodesians and their white allies may ultimately be able to take back the land. Similar suspicions of the AIDS epidemic as a biological warfare tool has been observed elsewhere in the world.[3]

Other local conspiracy allegations assume that larger global powers are somehow involved with the origin of the epidemic. Believers think of HIV as a biological weapon not specifically produced for use in Zimbabwe, but designed as a weapon for general use by global powers. Western countries have this terrible weapon to use in warfare against any group that hinders their access to wealth and power:

> HIV was used as biological warfare, created by the United States. I confidently believe that it was made intentionally to wipe out particular groups of people. HIV appeared during the war. It is said that the powder in the bullets and bombs contained the virus that causes AIDS.

These and comparable statements of interviewees reiterate that HIV was produced by Americans, and was then used by the Rhodesian forces as biological warfare by inserting the lethal agent into bullets and bombs. This view is the more surprising because the United States had nothing to do with the Rhodesian regime's attempt to remain in power. The United States had, in fact, opposed Rhodesian politics!

A logical extension of this argument would be to suspect white Zimbabweans or Great Britain, the former colonial power, of masterminding the conspiracy. This, however, happened only rarely. Mostly, white Americans were thought to be the conspirators.

The last quote presents a new idea, that "others" thought the land should be entirely cleansed of its residents. Some in Nkulumane expressed the view that HIV/AIDS is a plot to eradicate blacks. The goal of the epidemic is outright genocide. Usually they believe that this is done through secretly infecting people with HIV through individuals thought to be social deviants (for example, prisoners), or through encouraging deviant behavior (for example, through reading pornography, having sex with animals).

Regarding deviant individuals, some respondents believed that a malicious Western agency conspired against them:

Initially, people believed that the disease was brought to Africa by Americans and Britons to kill Africans. They sent former prisoners to Africa in order to spread the disease. These white prisoners were HIV-positive in order to infect blacks with the virus.

Such accounts are fostered by reports in the Zimbabwean media informing readers that an American laboratory artificially created the virus and tested it on volunteers—generally convicted prisoners—who were then released and sent to Africa (Anonymous 1986:36).

Regarding the encouraging of deviant behavior, some people suspected that Europeans arrived in Zimbabwe with their dogs. These Europeans then paid Zimbabwean women to sleep with the dogs, somehow resulting in HIV-infection. This narrative has been circulating for years and was known to most residents with whom I spoke. Other studies from Zimbabwe also report this narrative (Feldskov and Frederiksen 2000:24) and even far away areas such as West Africa knows variants of it (Machein 1999:43–48).

As in most conspiracy theories, individual informants add their own notions to the plot. They concur, however, that a white man, being the messenger of a group of conspirators, wanted to deliberately infect the women with HIV. From there the epidemic took its course, through sex among humans, causing many people to become infected with the virus, leading toward genocide. The conspiracy allegation, with its focus on bestiality, has strong moral connotations. Generally more people admit to believing in conspiracies with strong moral connotations than in general conspiracies such as the biological warfare theory. Immorality attaches to the acts of women who (presumably) took money for having sex with animals. The white conspirator used this moral deficiency for his purposes:

> Our people were having sex with dogs and being paid by white people. The whites did so because they wanted to use us blacks. They knew that we think all the time about money; we love money very much.

In other words, the white conspirator fulfills his evil plan because he is able to connect the plan to a local moral deficiency, the greed for money.

Another notion pertains to the nation's lack of moral leadership, which allows the conspiracy to happen. Had the political leadership been dedicated to the good of the nation, then AIDS would never have become such a threat to society:

> AIDS came indeed through a dog, at a time when President Mugabe was not around.

In discussion, people often criticized the president's frequent state visits out of the country. They implied that the country would be substantially better off if he had been more concerned with managing the country's affairs. Though the quote refers to the literal absence of the president, it implies his lack of moral leadership.

We see this and similar statements link the government's inadequate leadership to the AIDS epidemic. Similarly, these and other notions of morality allow us to interpret some AIDS conspiracy allegations as metaphors for the loss of morals and values. The function of sorcery beliefs, to teach and reinforce norms and values, may also apply to these conspiracy suspicions. Nevertheless, some people believe in the factual truth of an AIDS conspiracy.

This allows me to observe that informants expressed belief in various conspiracy beliefs despite their contradictions. If a malicious agent is indeed masterminding the eradication of blacks in order to get their land, then this agent will encounter a major problem in future. Who will work on the land? Large numbers of blacks would be needed as cheap labor. As analysts of conspiracy theories point out, conspiracy beliefs do not need to be coherent.

Other conspiracy theories solve such contradictions by arguing that some wicked agents plan to use HIV, not to totally eradicate blacks, but to limit their population. Views that assume an agent is preparing to change demographic patterns by limiting or lowering the numbers of the indigenous population have been unearthed in other parts of the world.[4] Such theories take into account the experience of Zimbabweans, that they are still a valuable asset in the white economy. They see that, though whites have owned land and factories, the overwhelming majority of the labor force has been black. The white conspirator will still need them after regaining land and political power.

Either outright genocide or population control of blacks is thought to be the final goal of the evil white agent. The presumed means of achieving these goals are presented in the following sections. Some of them are secretly achieved through programs established to benefit Zimbabweans, while others are outright poisoning of blacks in secret. They match numerous global legends about HIV/AIDS that focus on the contamination of objects and spaces (Goldstein 2004:39).

A central argument of interviewees was that deadly vaccines could achieve the goal of reducing the black population. Under the pretext of benevolence, an insidious plot is being executed. At times the actual vaccine is contaminated. In other cases residents were not so explicit; they just argued that vaccination campaigns caused those who were vaccinated to become ill:

> The whites are very "clever"; they tested many vaccines and medicines and found something to harm us. This harmful thing is used during immunizations and causes AIDS.

Again, as in other AIDS beliefs, the conspirators were "clever." Because medical professionals usually administer vaccines, these AIDS conspiracy allegations have some affinity to conspiracy suspicions directly implicating them. Here, however, the finger of blame is pointed at those organizing and masterminding vaccination campaigns, generally assumed to be whites in the West.

Suspicions pointing at vaccines are not new in Zimbabwe; for instance, in the 1960s a smallpox vaccination program and other preventive medical programs were compromised by a widespread belief among black Zimbabweans that they were means for whites to reduce the number of Africans (Kaler 1998:351). Similar reactions were later reported in relation to measles and malaria campaigns. Such historic suspicions became reactivated following reports in the international media that vaccination campaigns could have accidentally led to the AIDS epidemic, like one that a vaccine program resulted in the outbreak of AIDS in central

Africa (e.g., Wright 1987). People began to suspect a hidden plot behind campaigns that pretend to immunize but actually break down the human immune system through HIV. Similar reactions to vaccination and health programs were reported from other parts of the globe among subordinated and excluded racial and ethnic groups.

The vaccination conspiracy theory in Zimbabwe has an interesting twist. Several respondents argued that there actually is a powerful vaccine for HIV. The medical doctors have it, however they withhold it from black Zimbabweans. A belief that an available vaccine for HIV/AIDS is purposely being withheld is reported elsewhere in the world.[5] This belief is one of benign neglect, in contrast to other theories of malicious intent.

Other conspiracy beliefs are linked to contraceptives. Suspicions against contraceptives are not new in Zimbabwe and were reported particularly during the nationalist period before the country achieved majority rule (Kaler 1998:350, 2003; West 1994). Like the black population during the Rhodesian rule, other subordinated groups in many parts of the world have regarded birth control programs with suspicion, assuming that these are tools in the hand of the powerful to negatively impact the fertility and growth of the powerless.[6] The suspicion has been heightened globally in societies that place a strong emphasis on fertility—and when contraceptives alter gender relations.

Sometimes such contraceptive suspicions develop into conspiracy theories that a particular group is being kept from reproducing, thus severely curtailing the group's influence in society.[7] It should not come as a surprise that the experience of AIDS is interpreted in the light of such earlier suspicion. Because some devices used for family planning are also used to prevent transmission of HIV, existing suspicions easily get transferred to HIV/AIDS prevention campaigns. In many parts of the world, condoms are especially viewed with suspicion.

Some residents in Nkulumane believed that condoms are purposely distributed to infect people and thereby reduce their numbers. Reports on faulty condoms that originate from the West deepen such suspicions (Anonymous 1995; 1999c). When the local media report that condoms are not entirely safe, people argue that they represent some arcane danger. Particularly, in some Christian churches that oppose the use of condoms, these fears increase as reports grow more exaggerated. Sometimes they are worried by false information about the safety of condom use. This leads people to believe that the producers of condoms or some other malicious agent purposely added lethal HIV germs to condoms. Condom conspiracy allegations are widely known in Zimbabwe and other African countries.[8]

There is wide distribution of the suggested method to determine whether HIV is inside the condom. An informant told me that filling a condom with water and exposing it to sunlight caused "tiny worms," HIV germs, to become visible:

> The condom itself causes the disease. When you put water into condoms you will later see "tiny creatures" alive in them. When you use condoms, consequently these *amagciwane* enter the body. The producers of the condoms put *umuthi* into condoms; these are malicious people!

Stories like these have in common the assumption that a wicked agent has added HIV to the lubricant of the condoms. They use the local term *umuthi*, with its ambiguous meanings ranging from curative medicine to lethal poison, and its cognitive link to poisons used in sorcery practices. Sometimes the lubricant was assumed to be the *umuthi* that, much like traditional sorcery poisons, develops in the body to become the living HIV. At other times, the *umuthi* is believed to actually contain HIV, which is in the vernacular generally expressed with *isibungu* or *igciwane* (plural, *amagciwane*). The first term is a generic term for insects, worms, or other tiny creatures. The second term refers to invisible insects or agents causing disease, and is generally the vernacular expression for germs and viruses. The artist Shumba made a carving symbolically placing HIV on top of a couple, representing the fear of many couples of HIV-infection (page 152).

Common in such condom conspiracy allegations and other conspiracy suspicions implicating contraceptives is that they are perceived as Trojan horses, seemingly benevolent things, which, in fact, would kill or at least

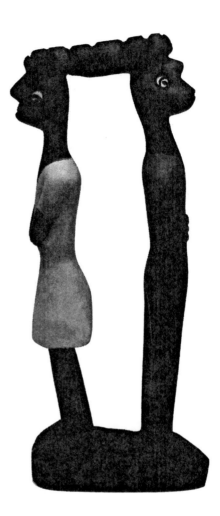

HIV in the indigenous imagination. (Carving by Sheunesu Shumba. Photo by Heinz Helf.)

harm Africans who used them (Kaler 1998:350). Conspirators pretend to be concerned with the well-being of people while they plot their death. And Western nations and agencies are the masterminds behind such plots.

AIDS contamination narratives actually appear to be more about moral discourse than about mechanisms of contracting the virus (Goldstein 2004:40; Webb 1997:148). The contaminated condom narrative is usually embedded in statements that condoms promote promiscuity and therefore AIDS (Pfeiffer 2004:79). It seems plausible to me that stories of contaminated condoms are, for some people with whom I spoke, actually metaphorical expressions of the danger of condom use because it is believed to promote promiscuity and therefore AIDS.

The belief that the condom is contaminated with HIV symbolizes the perceived danger of using a condom. Something with the condoms is dangerous; this may be HIV itself, or HIV may be just a metaphorical expression for something else regarded as dangerous, such as promiscuity. During interviews it became evident that many people closely associate condoms with promiscuity, which is viewed as risky. Such sexual behavior leads to a high risk for acquiring HIV. Accounts of the belief that condoms are contaminated are therefore metaphorical expressions of the danger of contracting HIV that sexual behavior represents. While some informants appear to believe in such a symbolic reading of the contaminated condom, others take quite literally the belief that condoms contain HIV.

Suspicions of AIDS conspiracies related to the poisoning of the food and water have been observed in various regions of the world[9] and were a central focus during my interviews in Zimbabwe. Even before HIV/AIDS appeared, food and water poisoning was always a major theme in conspiracy theories throughout history, and cross-culturally (Zukier 1987:98–99). Across the globe, the aim of such poisoning varies from inducing sterility to outright genocide.[10] Like other conspiracy suspicions, such narratives are historically embedded in an experience of subordination and exclusion that confers credibility upon them. Such conspiracy fears are also known in Zimbabwe.

In the 1970s a program to prevent cholera through treating the water supply was interpreted as a means of killing people by actually spreading cholera (Kaler 1998:351). During my fieldwork in 2003, nongovernmental organizations imported corn and millet from the United States. My informants in Nkulumane suspected that the imported flour might be poisoned "because Americans want to eradicate all blacks." Their suspicion of a food conspiracy echoes Ben Geer's *Something More Sinister*. White farmers in a Rhodesian pub are arguing:

As he started drinking his seventh gin of the night someone said, "Sterilize the munts![11] Put something in their mealie meal." (Geer 1998:215-216)

The quote from Geer's novel referred to the poisoning of corn flour, the main staple for most Zimbabweans. This reference is not farfetched, since Rhodesian forces were strongly suspected of using the poisoning of food (canned meat) as part of their military strategy (McGregor 1999:135, White 2004:224–25). These poisoned cans appeared again during my interviews:

AIDS is a thing of the whites. Indeed, they put it into our food. Otherwise how can someone old as me contract this disease! Especially the canned food is dangerous!

The legacy of the Rhodesian attempts to poison their enemies is that these attempts also "poisoned the future" (Brickhill 1992). Zimbabwean AIDS conspiracies not only involve poisoned cans of food but generally conclude that whites contaminated the food of black Zimbabweans with a poison that leads to AIDS, or even with the actual HIV virus.

Frequently, the poisoning agent is referred to as *umuthi*. Again, as in other conspiracy fears, the term *umuthi* indicates an affinity to sorcery practices, particularly the *isidliso* phenomenon, when substances used in sorcerous practices are added to food. This further supports the argument that the conspiracy complex has much in common with sorcery beliefs.

The accounts of various types of conspiracies are not the end of the story. The whites' plot backfired! The masterminds behind HIV did not anticipate that they would lose control over the epidemic, which then spread from the intended victims to mainstream society. Similar beliefs are reported elsewhere.[12]

Although some Zimbabweans admitted during interviews to a belief that HIV/AIDS is a plot against them as black Zimbabweans, or against blacks in general, they are aware that HIV/AIDS is not just a Zimbabwean issue or a continental issue; they know that HIV/AIDS is a global concern. Zimbabweans explain the fact that HIV/AIDS also affects non-black humans as an oversight on the part of those conspirators using HIV. Although their conspiracy aimed only at blacks in general, or black Zimbabweans in particular, they did not consider the further consequences of their plot. Yes, they are "smart" and "well-educated," but they are not so clever after all. They assumed an unbridgeable divide between blacks and whites, but did not consider that a white man could fall in love with a black girl and get infected. Despite efforts to set them apart, to divide them and prevent communication and intimacy on the same level, people of the different groups still meet and interact on all levels.

I am reminded of the movie *Gosford Park*, a social satire set in a 1930s English country estate (Altman 2001). On the surface, the aristocrats are wealthy and live comfortably, while the servants are just competent supporters, clearly separated from them. However, under the surface a morass of overlapping affairs is exposed; after all, both masters and servants are human. People pointed out during interviews that various connections between the races caused the evil AIDS plot to backfire:

> HIV was made by scientists in the laboratory, and they thought they would be able to control it. But at the end of the day they found out that it was uncontrollable. It happened that black and white had sexual intercourse and then the disease spread to all races. Whites are also dying of AIDS because they did not consider that a black person can fall in love with a white person. Sometimes it is not love but greed that brings them together. Whites thought that only they are rich and have money, but nowadays black people have money; and money is desired by everyone, black or white. And the white man now wanted to have the money from the black woman.

The quote refers to the conspirators' fundamental attitude, namely, greed. The conspirators are motivated by greed to plot against blacks using HIV/AIDS, a common feature in sorcery beliefs as well as conspiracy suspicions. But, greed is also the conspirators' downfall.

The conspirators engage in relations with their victims because they want the wealth of affluent black women; subsequently, they get infected with HIV. Greed made the whites blind and became the source of their own downfall. The moral message of this narrative is that those who conspired to plot the eradication of blacks will suffer the consequences. Those who plot genocide will not succeed but will suffer the same fate as the ones against whom they plotted.

Notes

1. From the wealth of accounts, I refer to three exemplary studies: Nicoll et al. 1993:234; Pipes 1997:5; and Tillotson and Maharaj 2001:95.

2. A "Freedom Fighter" is an individual who actively participated in the struggle to achieve majority rule.

3. See, for example Goertzel 1994: 734; Klonoff and Landrine 1999; and Thomas and Quinn 1991: 1499.

4. See, e.g., Levine and Ross 2002:12; Marcus 2002:90; and MacLean 1992.

5. Examples from other countries and regions are, e.g., du Toit 1965:59; and Knight 2000:153. That people in other countries hold a belief that an AIDS vaccine is purposely withheld is reported, e.g., by Karim 1993; and Tillotson and Maharaj 2001:94.

6. See, for instance, Nicoll et al. 1993:240; and Turner and Darity 1973.

7. This argument is, e.g., brought forward by Bird and Bogart 2003:264, 268; Guinan 1993:194; Makhobo 1989:20–21; Schneider and Fassin 2002:S49; and Simmons 2002:117.

8. See, for example, Chiroro et al. 2002:23–24, 30; Feldskov and Frederiksen 2000:23; McGrath 1992:67; Machein 1999:49–52; Marcus 2002:90; Nicoll et al. 1993:234; Pfeiffer 2004:94; Sabatier and Tinker 1988:96; Setel 1999:217, 240; Stadler 2003:363–64; Stally 2000:1; and Tillotson and Maharaj 2001:93–94. Though widely known, evidence of the actual distribution of conspiracy suspicions involving condoms widely differs in Africa and elsewhere from very high (e.g., Chiroro et al. 2002:23–24, 30) to very rare (e.g., Bogart and Thorburn 2005:216).

9. Typical examples are, e.g., Greunke 2001; Leclerc-Madlala 1997:364; Niehaus and Jonssen 2005:196; Tillotson and Maharaj 2001:94; and Turner 1993:137–44.

10. See, for example, Coombe 1997; Fenster 1999:72; Kelly 1995:64; Maines 1999:322; Parsons et al. 1999; Sasson 1995; Turner 1993:82–83; and Waters 1997.

11. *Munt* is a derogatory term used to speak about blacks. It is a derivative of *umuntu*, a term in many Bantu languages referring to a human being or an individual, particularly of black skin color. The plural in many languages is *abantu*.

12. See, for example, Goldstein 2004:96; Niehaus and Jonssen 2005:198; and Whetten-Goldstein and Nguyen 2002:173.

PART IV

The Implications of Culture

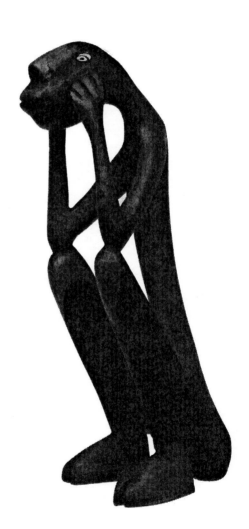

CHAPTER 9

Comparing Theories of Blame

In this book's journey through the colorful world of people's suspicions I have called attention to overlaps between conspiracy theories and sorcery beliefs. Though some studies refer to both, they do not explicitly compare and contrast them (e.g., Farmer 1992). Academic analysts have rarely looked simultaneously at conspiracy theories and sorcery arguments that were generated *within the same social setting*. These scholars may have assumed that conspiracy theories and sorcery beliefs are fundamentally distinct. Indeed, their relationship is usually described by dichotomous oppositions, e.g., Western vs. non-Western, modern vs. traditional, rational vs. magical (Sanders and West 2003:6–7). However, in the Zimbabwean case study I saw both types of explanatory models simultaneously, which allowed me to compare and contrast them within a single setting.

At first the evidence seemed to confirm that there are essential differences between the two types of causal explanation, such as the collective nature of the conspirator versus the individuality of the sorcerer, or the fact that victims of conspiracies are whole social groups while victims of sorcery are individuals.

A closer look lends some doubt to the conclusion that they are distinct phenomena. Although sorcery arguments draw more on inherited traditional beliefs and practices than conspiracy theories do, they also integrate aspects of contemporary life. Although conspiracy theories draw more on current events, they are also influenced by traditional thoughts and practices. Sorcery beliefs are an integral part of the *weltanschauung* of a people, but conspiracy suspicions are also part of the shared understanding about how the world works.

Because the two types of causal explanation have some patterns, structures, and functions in common, it is not surprising that they are frequently seen as a single category.[1] Further, society's misfortune is interpreted by individuals, who may explain their personal suffering through sorcery beliefs, which increases the potential for conflating the two categories (Loudon 1976:xi). This would explain the fact that during the Spanish influenza epidemic of 1918–1919 many Zimbabweans expressed their conviction that the whole country was "bewitched" (Shelley 1918).

Again and again my interviewees wove such overlaps and differences into one common narrative that most residents appear to believe: this story traces the origin of HIV/AIDS to an event during which some women reportedly had sexual intercourse with a dog. Strikingly similar versions of the narrative are reported from West Africa, where the story, as in Zimbabwe, was widely disseminated through the media (Machein 1999: 43–48).

The common denominator of the variations of this narrative is that some years ago, in an affluent Harare suburb, some women were paid by a white man to have sex with a dog. Many of my informants described this act as the origin of the AIDS epidemic in Zimbabwe. When I searched the National Archives in Harare, I found the original report, which appeared in 1991 on the front page of a national newspaper. Here is the gist of the original newspaper report:

> In what can be described as a bizarre and inhuman sex activity, police
> have confirmed the arrest of some women in Harare who were al-
> legedly indulging in sex with a dog in exchange for money. . . . The
> owner of the animal would screen[2] a video at each "sex session" whose

film-clips were allegedly destined for pornographic markets overseas. . . . The women were picked up at different times by the owner—believed to be a white man—at hotels and the Hellensdale Shopping Center in Borrowdale. . . . A former boyfriend of one of the dog's "mistresses" . . . said: "My former girlfriend confessed to me that she was having sex with a dog in exchange for money. She said this when I asked why a venereal disease I had contracted had taken four months to heal." . . . The women were understood to be shunning men in the suburb, saying they had better offers elsewhere. (Anonymous 1991g)

Although this news item purports to be based in fact, it was never fully substantiated, and later reports described it as "hearsay" (e.g., Anonymous 1991d). The veracity of the report is questionable because it suggests that the male dog got sexually aroused *on command*. Although male dogs may on occasion get sexually aroused by women, this hardly happens on command. It would be easier for a man to have sex with a female dog; in fact, acts of bestiality committed by men with various animals are reported from time to time in the local media (e.g., Anonymous 1990c, 1996b). My discussions with residents corroborate such reports.

Despite doubts about the truth of the report, numerous letters of outrage were published in both national and local newspapers.[3] In neither the original news report nor the letters that followed was HIV/AIDS mentioned—just an unnamed venereal disease thought to have come from the dog. The first mention of AIDS in connection with the dog narrative came later that same year (Gumbo 1991). Nevertheless, more than ten years later, my interviewees firmly linked the incident to the origin and spread of HIV/AIDS in Zimbabwe.

Narratives function as templates. They are malleable, and open to different interpretations. My informants developed different aspects of the dog narrative to express a particular argument. For some it took the form of a conspiracy theory. For others it took the form of a sorcery suspicion, a statement about morality, or something else. At times, residents' statements included lines of argument that are not logically connected and may even be contradictory. Some thought the dog narrative was both an account of a conspiracy and evidence of the decadence of society. The white man knowingly and deliberately used the dog to infect the women, but the women had had no qualms about having sexual intercourse with the animal. This mingling of accusations against malicious outsiders with accusations against immoral locals is typical of many of the sorcery beliefs and conspiracy theories presented in this book. The dog narrative is a prime example of both types of beliefs.

Some residents at the research site argued that the dog with which the women had sex was infected with HIV. They had identified the unknown disease of the original news story as HIV/AIDS. Such a reading of the narrative regards transmission by sexual contact as the start of the epidemic. That is, when the women were sleeping with this dog, they became infected and later spread the virus to others during sexual intercourse. From then on, the epidemic took its natural course.

Some respondents read this narrative as a morality tale. They argued that sexual intercourse between humans and animals is inappropriate and despicable. Humans simply should not engage in sexual encounters with animals. Similar remarks about incidents of bestiality were frequently expressed in print. Informants who agreed with a moral reading of this narrative tended to believe in a naturalistic origin of HIV: it mysteriously evolved when these women had sex with the dog, perhaps through the mingling of incompatible body fluids. Similar views, arguing that the disorderly mixing of animal and human blood caused AIDS, are extant in South Africa (Niehaus and Jonssen 2005:198).

Those who emphasize the moral dimension appear disinterested in the origin of HIV, arguing that immoral behavior *in general* results in AIDS. For them, the dog narrative is a metaphor about immorality and the actual existence of the dog is not important. Such informants wanted to emphasize that the AIDS epidemic is the result of immoral sexual behavior; frequently, the same informants went on to point out that it is those who engage in premarital or extramarital sexual intercourse who are the victims of AIDS. The explanation that sexual immorality is the cause of AIDS has nothing to do with either sorcery or conspiracy; it is a naturalistic, or moralistic, explanation of the epidemic.

Only after several months of fieldwork did I come to understand the metaphorical nature of my informants' expressions. One day a woman expressed her fear of bathing in icy water during the Zimbabwean winter by saying "There is a crocodile looking at you from the water." Listening to her, I suddenly realized that my interviewees customarily used metaphor to express their fears. The oft-repeated remark that condoms are contaminated with HIV, for example, metaphorically expresses a more complex set of ideas: that condoms are dangerous because they encourage promiscuity, promiscuity leads to HIV infection, and those who encourage the use of condoms are exposing us to a high risk of infection. Obviously the dog narrative could also be a metaphorical expression. However, while some meant such expressions metaphorically, others took them literally.

Three distinct lines of thought can be identified in the interviews that mentioned the sex between the women and the dog. First, some informants emphatically maintained that this man knew the women would get infected with HIV when they had sex with his dog. He knowingly allowed it, showing no human concern for the women who were at risk of becoming infected with the deadly virus.

Second, other informants argued that he had conducted a medical experiment with the dog, injecting it with HIV before he paid the women to have sex with it. He was, they thought, curious about how long the virus needs to incubate until AIDS develops. The women were human guinea pigs in this bizarre experiment.

Third, still others attributed an even more sinister motivation to the white man: he deliberately infected them with HIV in order to harm not only them but also everyone with whom they subsequently had sex. In other words, his aim was to kill, and the women were just a means to that end.

That the owner of the dog is believed to be a white man is important; some informants concluded that he represents all whites who are out to harm or even kill blacks. HIV/AIDS is a tool in white hands to get rid of blacks, perhaps because whites think that there are too many blacks in the country, or because they simply despise blacks, or because they want something from them. Generally respondents believed that the motive was the acquisition of land, a highly politicized issue in Zimbabwe.

The conspiratorial nature of these theories does not exhaust their meanings. This dog story is as much a sorcery suspicion as it is a conspiracy theory. The white owner of the dog, the conspirator, could easily be called a sorcerer in traditional contexts, and the dog as a means for implementing his conspiracy could be seen as a sorcerer's familiar. The aims of the conspiracy are also typical goals of sorcery, namely to inflict harm on the intended victims and to gain some profit from their suffering.

Informants defined a sorcerer mainly in terms of motivation: a sorcerer is anyone who knowingly and deliberately plots to inflict harm on one or more individuals. The specifics are of secondary importance. The tendency of an individual to do evil may be either social or idiosyncratic in nature. This issue touches the core of Evans-Pritchard's distinction between the inborn trait of a witch and the learned trait of a sorcerer. The tendency to inflict harm may be due to an inherited trait running in the sorcerer's kinship group that endows the sorcerer with certain evil power and knowledge. Some kin-groups are known to be malicious, causing difficulties for those with whom they deal. This is sometimes expressed through saying that *balemimoya emibi* (they have evil spirits). The term can refer to a literal spirit possession or be metaphorical in the sense of having an innately evil disposition. Both usages were implied by informants.

Alternately, the tendency to aggression may be due not to family influence but to an individual's evil desire that is unrelated to kinship. Such an individual actively pursues knowledge of inflicting harm and is individually to blame. The tendency to aggression is a learned character trait, so it can be said that this person *ulomoya omubi* (has an evil spirit). While this term could also refer to literal possession by an evil spirit, it is generally metaphorical when the individual is at fault.

The inclination to inflict harm is not exclusively linked to sorcery practices such as *isidliso* and *ulunyoka*, and it is clear that anyone—even whites, who would not know traditional sorcery—can show this inclination. Whites *balomoya omubi* (have a bad spirit), an expression that people interpreted in ways similar to the earlier ones; that is, a white man may be inherently evil or may have learned to be evil.

Some informants argued that all whites want to inflict harm and are therefore sorcerers. Their tendency to aggression is inherent—this is just how they are! In contrast, other informants, aware of differences in whites' attitudes toward Africans, argue that some whites have basically benevolent attitudes and behavior while other whites appear to be malevolent, particularly against Africans. The latter are then like sorcerers, who have somehow learned this tendency to aggression. In other words, as is true of Africans, inflicting harm is not something inherited through descent, but actively acquired. Both understandings of the origins of aggression, generationally transmitted or individually acquired, were applied to the whites and other collective conspirators.

The dog story allows another comparison between conspiracy and sorcery if we look at the white man's means of inflicting harm. The owner of the dog knew that having sex with his animal would either create the virus or transmit the existing virus from the dog to humans. HIV was the tool through which he intended to inflict harm—the means to implement his conspiracy.

However, HIV can also be interpreted through the sorcery paradigm. HIV was like the *umuthi*, harmful "medicine" through which a sorcerer attempts to hurt others. Just as a traditional sorcerer prepares or obtains concoctions, poisons, and charms, the *umuthi* of HIV serves the specific goal of causing suffering to the unsuspecting victim. Consequently, the white man in the dog narrative can be called a sorcerer. He used HIV as a traditional sorcerer would use *umuthi*: secretly administering poison to an unknowing and unsuspecting victim. Even if the targeted victims did not trust whites, they were not likely to have suspected something sinister.

HIV is hidden, difficult to detect, like any sorcery poison. It is similarly difficult to identify sorcerers, particularly those who acquire knowledge in order to inflict harm. Even those sorcerers from descent groups known to have sorcerer members are not easy to identify despite the vigilance of their potential victims; they are still able to inflict harm secretly. Unless a person assumes that all whites are evil, it is difficult to decide who is dangerous. To sum up, both the sorcery and the conspiracy paradigms imply that there is more than meets the eye. There are hidden and malicious forces at work using hidden means to inflict harm. The introduction of HIV can be interpreted by both the sorcery and conspiracy paradigms.

Another connection in the dog story between sorcery and conspiracy is that the white man had an explicit economic interest. Both types of belief are connected to the illicit accumulation of wealth through inflicting harm and causing suffering (Moore and Sanders 2001:11–18). Recall that the *ondofa*, the sorcerers' familiars, collect money and other material goods for their owners. In the original dog narrative, the white man videotaped the sexual encounter, reportedly to sell it on the Western market. He not only deliberately inflicted harm and subsequent death on his victims but also planned to profit from his action. A central theme of many of the conspiracy theories described in this book was that someone profited from deliberately infecting people with HIV. As mentioned earlier, acquiring land was thought to be the ultimate goal for the conspirators. Both the sorcerer and the conspirator wanted to profit from their victims' suffering and death. In other words, the white man can be seen both as a sorcerer and a conspirator.

But what about the women who slept with the dog? They also profited from the sexual encounter; the white man is believed to have paid them exceptionally well. Are the women thought to be sorcerers in the traditional sense, or conspirators in a more modern sense? A clue to the answer comes from the dog's presence in the story. As mentioned earlier when discussing theories of medical experiments, sex with animals in general, and dogs in particular, is viewed as highly immoral. Only extreme social deviants would sleep with dogs.

Actually, in southern Africa sorcerers are thought to sleep with their familiars, mainly monkeys, baboons, and dogs (Brain 1975:186). The dog in our narrative could be seen as a sorcerer's familiar and the women sleeping with the dog as sorcerers, although subordinate to the white sorcerer. Supporting this line of thought, informants agreed that the prime motivation for sex with the dog was greed. Greed was, in fact, generally assumed by residents to be one of the prime movers for sorcery. In the original news report, the women who slept with the dog were said to shun men afterward because they had "better offers elsewhere" (that is, it was more profitable to sleep with the dog). The question is, should they be viewed primarily as sorcerers or as victims of the white sorcerer?

166

Excerpts, first from a local newspaper report and then from one of my interviews, suggest an answer:

> It is unfortunate that a male member of society contracted a venereal disease from one of these prostitutes—maybe the appropriate term is "bitch" in this case, since a dog is involved. (Gumbo 1991)

> The woman slept with the dog. But the woman was a real bitch! She slept later with men too!

Zimbabweans are aware of the two meanings of the English word *bitch* and used it to comment on the narrative. For them the women were morally wrong but still victims of an intentional plot, whether an act of sorcery or a conspiracy. If someone could be called a sorcerer, then it is the white man. For them, the women may have been "greedy bitches" but not "wicked witches."

The dog story illustrates a link between this conspiracy narrative and sorcery. Zimbabweans observe that canine sexuality is extraordinarily uncontrolled, and driven by instinct, the opposite of human behavior, which is guided by norms and values. Chapter 5 related that, in some forms of *ulunyoka,* sorcerers use the genitals of dogs to provoke the same sexual behavior in victims (Zhakata 1992). The dog narrative could simply mean that the white man engaged his victims in uncontrolled sexual behavior that carries a high risk of acquiring HIV; there does not necessarily have to be a real dog involved. Such a reading of the narrative comes close to a metaphorical interpretation; the dog simply represents the fact that immoral women were paid by someone to have sex, engaged in uncontrolled sexual intercourse, and became infected with HIV.

This brings us back to the Zimbabweans moralistic interpretation of the origin of the AIDS epidemic—that HIV/AIDS is so widespread because of prostitution and uncontrolled sex. Nuances of the sorcery and conspiracy complexes express these notions. Like sorcery beliefs, conspiracy theories may foster solidarity and collective action. Both types have a strong moral undertone. They function to reinforce the social values and norms of a group by describing the opposite, and are intended to promote social cohesion.[4] While some informants appeared to follow this line of argument, others opted for a literal reading of the narrative in terms of both the sorcery and the conspiracy paradigms.

The dog narrative illustrates that the dividing line between sorcery and conspiracy accusations can be blurred. However, despite some parallels, there are fundamental differences between conspiracy suspicions and sorcery arguments. As we have seen, sorcery is invoked in order to explain hardship inflicted on an individual or a small group of related people (Kluckhohn 1944:71). In contrast, conspiracy theories are more commonly invoked to explain collective woes, explaining why larger social, regional, ethnic, racial, or other groups encounter misfortune.

A further difference between the two causal explanations is related to how the insidious plot is implemented. Conspirators are assumed to work in groups. In other words, a conspiracy of one is no conspiracy at all (Keeley 1999:116; Moscovici 1987:155). The collective nature of conspiracies underlies the term itself, derived from *conspirare*, to "blow," "sound," or "breathe together" (Zonis and Joseph 1994:449). Indeed, conspiracy beliefs are suspicions of crimes plotted by one group against another group (Zukier 1987:93, 98).

Consequently, if the white culprit in the dog narrative is seen as representing evil whites who are out to destroy blacks, then the story is a conspiracy suspicion. If, however, the white individual planned and implemented his plot alone, and wanted to profit from using only the women whom he had paid to have sex with the dog, then the story is a sorcery accusation. Both usages of the dog narrative were evident during my discussions with Zimbabweans.

Another evident distinction between sorcery beliefs and conspiracy theories is the identification of the culprit as insider or outsider. People think sorcerers are close to the victim, perhaps family members (of a different lineage, such as a wife) or a neighbor, or a colleague at work. In this case the sorcerer is an insider, albeit a troublemaking insider. We could say the sorcerer is an insider-outsider. In contrast, conspirators are generally total strangers, perhaps foreigners, whites, or highly educated and wealthy individuals. In this case the conspirator is an outsider-outsider. The "other" blamed for sorcery is the malevolent intimate, while the "other" blamed for conspiracy is the malevolent stranger.[5] Thus, the dog narrative fits the conspiracy paradigm better than the sorcery paradigm.

Another major difference is that sorcery arguments, unlike the typical conspiratorial model, tend to follow closely known patterns and ingredients. Thus, a sorcerer uses certain herbs, prepares these in a traditional manner, and administers them correctly in order to be effective. Sorcery practices tend to be closely informed by tradition. Conspiracy theories look beyond the traditional to the scientific. American biological warfare laboratories, contraceptives, food additives, and more are seen as tools to implement a conspiracy. The whites are "clever"; they know how to produce things in their laboratories and factories and transport them secretly to harm their victims. When the narrative posits an artificially manufactured virus that is injected into a dog, then it is more akin to a conspiracy allegation.

The dog complex is atypical in that it combines both conspiracy and sorcery elements. Most other theories that surfaced during interviews fit better in either the sorcery or the conspiracy category.

A further question remains to be answered: When will sorcery or conspiracy theories be invoked? These theories are now on the cultural "menu" of Zimbabweans and people elsewhere. Sorcery is a traditional thought pattern available to virtually everyone. Conspiracy theories circulate widely. The fact that these thought patterns are extant does not, however, explain why some adopt them and others do not.

Most of those who accept sorcery or conspiracy beliefs are also fully aware of the sexual nature of AIDS. So, how are people able to combine their knowledge of sexual transmission with beliefs in the causation of sorcery or conspiracy. My interview data indicate that, in the same conversation, informants were able to shift from marital infidelity to poverty and then to foreigners or sorcery as causes for the AIDS epidemic. Such

City Life   Boyd Maliki

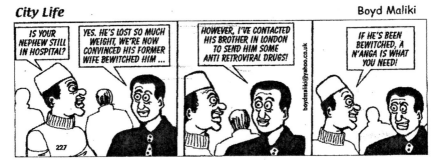

Harare Daily News, January 31, 2003.

shifts in argument show up in all sets of data and leave the researcher wondering about the foundation of such reasoning. This conflicted pattern is reflected in a cartoon that appeared in one of the local newspapers (above). How can people be aware of the sexual origin of AIDS and still invoke other causes? Is this not a contradiction?

Not really. Human beings are masters of causal ambiguity and creativity. Anthropology and other social sciences may attempt to find why one explanation is selected over another, but such attempts should be wary of an overly systematized view of the way people think. I observed that, for many Zimbabweans, the AIDS issue was not a question of this theory or that theory. Many expressed a number of contradictory theories simultaneously and oscillated between them. Similar observations have been made elsewhere (e.g., de Blécourt 1999:213)

At least for some people with whom I spoke, this phenomenon can be explained through what I call "thinking out loud." The questions asked by me or my assistants caught them off guard; they had not yet developed an opinion about the causation behind the AIDS epidemic and they listed all kinds of theories that appeared credible to them. Because HIV/AIDS is so prevalent at the research site, impacting all households in one way or another, no single explanation would be adequate across the board.

In simultaneously recognizing the operation of a variety of conflicting factors, the townspeople of Zimbabwe showed a sophistication similar to those of great philosophers, who also concerned themselves with causal exploration. For instance, Aristotle distinguished between two pairs of causes.[6] The first pair works internally and consists of (1) formal causes, which operate through the form internal to the organism, and (2) material causes, which are the way that the matter of a thing affects it. The second pair refers to external causation and consists of (1) the final causes, which pull the organism toward its final perfection, and (2) efficient causes, which work among objects to move or change them. In other words, great philosophers recognize, like the townspeople of Zimbabwe, the ambiguous and hierarchically nested structure of causality.

For an anthropologist and his informants, the latter type of causality—efficient causality through visible external factors—is more interesting. Thomas Aquinas adopted this theory of the four causes and argued that there is a distinction between different kinds of efficient causes: the pre-existing (primary) efficient and the intermediate (secondary) efficient causes.[7] Similar distinctions have been applied in the medical sciences. Medical historians find that the understanding of disease in medicine has traditionally been multidimensional (Phillips 1990:138; Porter 1993:1458). More specifically, Pelling notes that explicit distinctions comparable to those of the great philosophers were used by medical scientists to conceptualize the etiology of disease:

> Classical philosophy and epistemology made available to medicine an elaborate structure of explanation involving a hierarchy of causes. *First or primary causes* were cosmological or divine. . . . *Remote causes* related to the state of the atmosphere, or influences . . . broad enough in scope to bring about the rise and fall of epidemics. . . . *Immediate causes* related primarily to the more local environment or experiences of the diseased person. . . . *Predisposing causes* could overlap with this category but were also invoked to cover characteristics of the individual's life or heredity that might render him or her usually liable to a given disease. *Proximate causes* came closest to defining the diseased state or process occurring in the diseased body. . . . It should be stressed that an agent in one category of cause could be seen as also belonging to, or changing into, another category, as a result of a given set of circumstances. Causes could act singly or in concert in any given instance of disease. (Pelling 1993:312)

Anthropologists similarly distinguish between ultimate and the immediate/instrumental/proximate causes of an illness (Carneiro 1977:222; Green 1999:41–42). Applied to the AIDS epidemic, this means that AIDS can be regarded both as natural and supernatural; you can get it from another person who is infected and you can get it through sorcery (Farmer 1992:101–104). Zimbabweans (and, presumably, people elsewhere) have the same perception of hierarchically nested causality that philosophers such as Aristotle and Aquinas elaborate in more abstract language. People understand that there may be, particularly in mysterious situations, causes nested within causes.

In my research, people almost always asserted that the immediate cause of HIV/AIDS is through sexual contact or (less frequently expressed) through blood or bodily fluids. While recognizing these immediate causes, however, my informants also recognize less visible, more remote causes. People need an explanation for the presence of the illness in the blood that is usually transmitted sexually. How did the illness first get into the Zimbabwean bloodstream?

When secondary remote causes are invoked here they in no way deny the importance of sexual transmission. There may be a malicious agent who deliberately manufactured HIV, someone who used his HIV-infected dog to infect humans, or someone who contaminated condoms with HIV. These more remote causes (which Aquinas and other philosophers have labeled as primary, but which anthropologists would label as remote and secondary) may also include poverty or an oppressive government that creates the conditions which shape unsafe sexual behavior. This list of remote secondary causes includes sorcerers who "own" sexually hyperactive familiars that rape and infect humans, or ancestors who withdraw their protection from their descendents who subsequently get infected with HIV.[8] It is possible to point to these remote secondary causes and attribute responsibility for AIDS to others or to certain conditions, while at the same time fully acknowledging the individual's responsibility for HIV/AIDS.

It would be absurd to attribute these notions of hierarchically nested causality to the entire Zimbabwean population. There are some who doubt that HIV/AIDS exists. For them AIDS is not a newly occurring illness but one in existence throughout human history that can be interpreted through the sorcery paradigm. The wasting of the body is thought to be due to *isidliso*, poisons added to the food, or to *ulunyoka*, the magical poison harming the lover of a married woman, or even due to being maltreated by a sorcerer's familiar, the *undofa*.

But such people who deny the reality of AIDS are in a minority. Some, in fact, may do so in reaction to the stigma of HIV/AIDS and the hopelessness that a terminal disease represents. Most of my informants were fully aware that AIDS is both recent and real. Their explanations for this lethal new phenomenon implicitly incorporated the hierarchically nested causal models: sexual transmission is the immediate cause by which individual X, Y, or Z gets AIDS, but the path to this vulnerability has been created by the operation of more remote causes, including conspiracy, sorcery, political irresponsibility, and poverty. My informants are not philosophers. But in searching for the causes of AIDS, they base their causal models on the same assumptions of hierarchically nested causality pursued by the philosophers, nuanced models by which remote secondary causes pave the way for the operation of the immediate, primary vehicle of sexual transmission.

Notes

1. This argument is brought forward, e.g., by Groh 1987:4; Jacques-Chaquin 1987:82–83; and Stevens 1996:1228. Pipes' distinction (1996:10–11, 21–22) between small-scale conspiracies by a single or a few agents and large-scale conspiracies involving a network of individuals aspiring to acquire major influence could allow the incorporation of sorcery beliefs—essentially small-scale conspiracies—within the conspiracy paradigm, at least in the southern African context.

2. "Screening" means here to "tape" or "film" the event.

3. From the many letters, the following are typical examples: Anonymous 1991e; Chamakuhwa 1991; Makuve 1991; and Mathe 1991.

4. This has been argued for conspiracy theories, e.g., by Abalakina-Paap et al 1999:638; Berlet 1997; Beauvois and Joule 1998; Festinger 1957; Fine 1992:24; Pipes 1996:300–305; Robins and Post 1997:55, 93; and Sasson 1995:278. For a comparable argument for sorcery see, e.g., Beidelman 1963:96–97 and Kluckhohn 1944:113. See also: Harmon-Jones 2000:185–89.

5. For this argument in relation to the two types of belief, see, e.g., Darling 1999:734; Farmer 1992:230–43; Geschiere 1998: 815; Hellinger 2003; Niehaus and Jonssen 2005:203; Schoepf 2001:341–42; and Treichler 1999:220–26.

6. Aristotle offers his general account of the four causes in the third treatise of the second book of *Physics* (Aristotle 1934), as well as in the second treatise of the fifth book of *Metaphysics* (Aristotle 1933).

7. Thomas Aquinas discusses the theory of the four causes in the treatise on the creation in his *Summa Theologica*, Question 44 (Thomas Aquinas 1947) as well as in the first book of the *Summa Contra Gentiles* (Thomas Aquinas 1975).

8. One category of supernatural causation for HIV/AIDS referred to ancestral causation, which I have described elsewhere (Rödlach 2005).

CHAPTER 10

Applications for the AIDS Crisis

I have discussed the theoretical issues that arose as I compared sorcery with conspiracy suspicions, two types of causal explanations that are neither identical nor neatly separated. Both are theories that attribute blame for misfortune to a villainous "other." Because they have similarities, each can foster the development of the other, not just in Zimbabwe but across cultures. People who resort to them are trying to make sense of the AIDS epidemic through nested causality and shifting discourses.

This study of sorcery and conspiracy as they relate to the AIDS epidemic has implications beyond academia. My professional filter is that of anthropology, a discipline that carves out patterns across cultures and frames them within theoretical models to better understand the human experience. But staying within the confines of a single analytical perspective limits the interpretation of data. Throughout this book I have adopted various theoretical stances in order to reveal the colorful diversity of AIDS conjectures in Zimbabwe and elsewhere.

The methodological guidelines I used to investigate AIDS in Zimbabwe are applicable to other epidemics. Because people hide their true beliefs about the origins of misfortune, studies are difficult, but researchers need to collect reliable information about beliefs in order to draw valid conclusions. An important first step is to select methods designed to establish a trust relationship between data collectors and informants. Trust is important in any study—but it is crucial when researchers inquire into sensitive issues.

When individuals respond to a researchers' probing, they say only what is on their mind at the moment, not necessarily including every thought they have had on the subject! Researchers need to pose the same questions at different times and in different situations; only then will they be able to construct a reasonably complete picture. Over time, researchers are able to identify associations between people's beliefs and the conditions shaping their lives.

Another complication of sensitive research is the way in which moral judgments are interwoven with attitudes toward both sorcery and conspiracy. When people talk about the origin of misfortune, they often do so indirectly, in metaphorical terms. Recall that metaphors are implied comparisons in which the speaker likens one thing to another as if they were the same, thus referring to something beyond the literal meaning. Zimbabweans used sorcery and conspiracy suspicions as vehicles to express their views about the behavior of certain individuals, the conduct of particular groups, and the state of society in general. Moral valuations were at the core of such views.

It is also essential to listen carefully, because it is not easy to determine if an informant means a statement literally or metaphorically. The same expression can have different meanings, depending on the speaker's personality and on local usage. We have seen this throughout the book, and in particular detail during my analysis of the dog narrative.

To understand people's views, we need to address the setting and the familiar thought patterns: sorcery and conspiracy suspicions need to be contextualized. That is a common strategy in a holistic discipline like anthropology. People's AIDS beliefs match their experience in other dimensions of their life. Thus I studied the historic, political, and economic aspects of Zimbabwean life, as well as common thought patterns such as blaming dynamics, to demonstrate the impact these conditions have had on AIDS beliefs. When these conditions change, perceptions of the AIDS epidemic will change. This is true not only for the Zimbabwean study but also for any study of AIDS beliefs.

We have seen that the two types of causal explanation discussed in this book—sorcery and conspiracy suspicions—are disseminated and evolve through specific vehicles. The media and the government play instrumental roles in formulating conspiracy theories and it would be useful if researchers were to investigate their influence.

We have demonstrated that only long-term research and repeated data collection from the same individuals can reliably discover what people actually believe. The long-established method of participant observation, however, is threatened by time and funding constraints. Researchers are forced by a competitive job market to complete their studies quickly and to publish at once; funding agencies are receiving less public and private monies and disburse their scarce funds sparingly; and the contractual and logistic constraints of consulting, where increasing numbers of anthropologists find work, force them to come up with data and recommendations as early as possible (Manderson and Aaby 1992; Beebe 1995; Bennett 1995; Spittler 2001:22). The ideal of a whole year of fieldwork (excluding the period of learning the local language) that covers a full cycle of the seasons may soon be only a footnote in anthropological history, which would compromise the quality of our research, particularly when we study issues of such a sensitive nature as sorcery and conspiracy.

This study has pragmatic implications. Anthropology has always served practical purposes—including some of which we are not so proud. Professionals have applied the skills and knowledge gained during training and research to the solution of social problems whenever possible. The rapidly growing field of applied anthropology indicates the increasing importance of this dimension of anthropology.

In the Introduction I distinguished between *disease* and *illness*. This distinction points up the fact that perceptions about the causes of HIV/AIDS, how to deal with its symptoms, and how to treat it may differ widely among social groups, and between social groups and those attempting to ameliorate their suffering. Awareness of widely held AIDS illness beliefs may determine the success or failure of prevention programs and whether care of those suffering full-blown AIDS can be improved. If popular AIDS beliefs are not known to healthcare providers, then health professionals will be unable to direct their messages successfully to the individuals they want to assist, with potentially disastrous consequences for their health and that of society. If healthcare personnel cannot communicate adequately with those they hope to serve, that failure may foster suspicion, including the inference that providers have been instrumental in the spread of the AIDS epidemic. People do not develop trust of "outsiders" who seem to lack genuine care or a willingness to listen to concerns (see also Sabatier 1987:121). Caretakers with preconceived ideas and a distant approach may actually encourage the development of conspiracy theories.

Chapter 6 offered an example of healthcare providers who did not connect their AIDS messages with the beliefs that people were developing and expressing. Providers tended to ignore the Zimbabweans' strong interest in the origin of HIV, so people looked for answers elsewhere and found them in reckless statements of local politicians and sensationalistic news reports. People developed their own beliefs about the causes of AIDS, in contrast to the cause healthcare providers were promoting: irresponsible sexual behavior.

A generally accepted cause was not sex with an HIV-positive individual but the workings of a sorcerer or conspirator. Thus, the high risk of HIV transmission during sexual intercourse was relegated to secondary importance. Further, people's suspicions discouraged them from protecting themselves when engaging in high-risk sexual intercourse because they had concluded that condoms were contaminated with HIV. Healthcare professionals might have persuaded people to engage in responsible sexual behavior had they addressed their beliefs about the origin of AIDS. Having said that, I must repeat the cautionary note from the previous chapter, namely, that peoples' attention to sorcery and conspiracy does not necessarily mean they ignore the sexual transmission of HIV. But we cannot deny that such suspicions lead some people to downplay sexual means of HIV-infection and to engage in high-risk sexual behavior.

Sexual behavior is, of course, influenced by other factors too numerous to discuss here. My observations indicate that the desperate economic condition of many families cause people to lose sight of HIV/AIDS. Their concern is not a disease that has an incubation period of several years; their concern is to have sufficient food on the table today and to pay the month's bills. HIV/AIDS is far beyond the time frame they see as realistic for their life. Many people said that AIDS is the least of their concerns because, by the time full-blown AIDS develops, they will already be dead of starvation.

A complex array of factors influence people's sexual behavior; sorcery and conspiracy suspicions are just two of them. Healthcare providers need to be aware of these factors and views, to address people's concerns, and to respond by incorporating them in their programs. The result will be more appropriate strategies to prevent new HIV-infections and to improve the care for those who already have AIDS.

During my years in Zimbabwe I spoke with a number of health professionals who took people's concerns seriously and used them as a starting point for discussions about curbing the spread of AIDS. I felt uneasy, however, with agencies whose priorities were elsewhere. They set up costly organizational structures, implemented strategies fabricated in some faraway headquarters, and then gave their backers numerical indicators of the programs' efficiency. I do not doubt their genuine intentions but I saw the ineffectiveness of their strategies. Funds for HIV/AIDS awareness and prevention programs—as well as initiatives to care for AIDS sufferers—would have been better spent if agency representatives had first sat down with people, learned their language, got to know their joys, fears, and hopes, and only then designed intervention and care programs. Instead, agencies tend to implement their prefabricated programs without much concern about whether they are grounded in people's fears, concerns, and interests.

To illustrate, I offer my observations of a local AIDS agency, one that represents a wide range of governmental and non-governmental agencies, healthcare providers, and others working in the field of AIDS awareness, prevention, and care. This particular AIDS agency is funded mainly by overseas organizations and has established headquarters in the center of Bulawayo, the Zimbabwean city where I did my fieldwork. The agency aims at promoting and supporting AIDS programs, both in the city and in the two provinces of Matabeleland. Its representatives visit and encourage AIDS groups, in the township and beyond, to implement a wide variety of AIDS programs; they organize AIDS awareness events throughout the city either independently or in conjunction with smaller local groups; they publish posters and leaflets with AIDS messages; they report in the local news; they maintain a small library with literature on the epidemic; and they offer testing and counseling in their headquarters. At a first glimpse, the agency's contributions seem impressive.

A closer look raises some doubts about the actual influence of the agency locally. There is a startling gap between the agency's infrastructure and visibility in the township and its cooperation with local efforts. Headquarters staff have vehicles so they can reach destinations quickly, and offices are furnished with top-quality office equipment. The agency frequently organizes workshops for their workers and collaborators in fancy hotels. The staff seem to earn decent salaries and are provided with amenities far beyond the reach of many Zimbabweans. This liberal spending for infrastructure and employees starkly contrasts with the downscale support the agency offers to programs in the townships. I give two examples.

I met a teacher in Nkulumane township who had established an AIDS awareness program for primary school children. The program included, among other things, singing and sports competitions between township schools and peer education after school. This teacher lamented that they had had to cancel the program due to lack of funding. The AIDS agency had stopped contributing to this program, which was modest in comparison to the cost of running the stylish agency office but crucial for the township. A successful, locally developed AIDS awareness program for children, previously attracting hundreds of them and engaging them throughout weeks of preparation, could not be continued due to lack of funds. This low-cost event that involved a whole community had a substantially larger impact on AIDS prevention than some of the programs developed by overseas philanthropists with the help of expatriate consultants.

A second example is that of a township group of adults and adolescents who were actively responding to the epidemic. Despite financial constraints, they established programs for school children with music, dance, and theatrical performances; they engaged local healers, nurses, and medical doctors to discuss the local response to the epidemic and to plan efforts for curbing the spread of the disease; they provided modest financial support for households suffering from the effects of the epidemic; and they counseled those suffering from full-blown AIDS. However, these humble efforts did not go far, due to the minimal funding the group received from the AIDS agency.

These two examples illustrate the contrast between the superior infrastructure established by many AIDS agencies and their inferior funding for actual projects. Zimbabweans understood the contrast between the façade and the lack of funding; they said that representatives of such agencies *bayatsheba lenyama kokuphela, thina siyatsheba letswayi kuphela* (eat meat all the time, while our relish is just salt!). A Zimbabwean said that many AIDS agencies make no difference in people's lives—that hardly anyone would notice if they ceased to operate. Many of my informants said they did not feel that helping them was a priority of some AIDS agencies.

I do not want to blame such situations solely on employees of AIDS agencies. Many of them have simply learned to play by the rules of their organizations, which come with preconceived ideas about how an AIDS agency has to be operated. Let's face it, these agencies provide a means of generating income for the families of their employees. One could say that, in addition to the public and the private sector, the AIDS sector has become a major source of income for some Zimbabwean households.

At times the widespread perception that AIDS agency workers live well off these organizations turns into anger. Having been confused with an AIDS agency worker, one of my assistants was thrown out of a house by the angry owner, who accused him of "eating well" from AIDS funds while AIDS sufferers continue without much support. The approach of following preconceived ideas when setting up an agency must be blamed for creating a local "AIDS bourgeoisie."

Following preconceptions is responsible for another fundamental problem—that representatives of the agencies are detached from the people for whom their agency should make a difference. The healthcare providers' detachment from the people has consequences pertinent to the theme of this book. This lack of personal involvement with the people results in a gap between people's beliefs and the messages the agencies disseminate. I jotted down AIDS slogans and poster messages in Zimbabwe, including those emanating from the headquarters of the AIDS agency under our scrutiny. Generally, these messages are in line with international AIDS programs but lack local flavor.

Local messages are strikingly absent in agency pronouncements, but I found them in clinics, churches, and other places where people meet. They were often entirely different from the agency messages, and were printed with a local design or even produced by hand. At times, I came across people in the township who used the agency's posters and leaflets but had written over images and text to "correct" the messages. People's interest in AIDS was evident, but their concerns and responses to the epidemic were not always in line with what AIDS agencies and other healthcare providers did (Manderson 1998). There is a gap between their clients' understandings and those of some AIDS agencies. Why? Perhaps because AIDS agency workers and health professionals look more to satisfying their backers than to the needs of the people they are supposed to serve.

This widespread pattern is fostered by the attitude that it is not necessary to "learn" from people who face the consequences of the AIDS epidemic daily. Many agencies already "know" what needs to be done; they have been told what to do by their overseas backers and expatriate consultants and don't want to "waste" time by talking with people (Good 1994). No wonder that people's views of the epidemic are not a match with agencies' views.

I was with a group of HIV-positive individuals who met regularly to support each other. One of their counselors, a member of the agency we are scrutinizing, a youngish and trendy-looking woman, regularly stormed into their weekly meeting, talking to them in a rush, and then drove off in her fancy car, leaving a cloud of dust behind. But nothing else. I was told that this is the way she usually comes and goes. She does not take time to sit down with people, listen to their stories, and discuss strategies for implementing AIDS care and prevention with them. Yet, in the reports of the AIDS agency to its backers, this local group of HIV-positive individuals is listed as one of their success stories. Because this case is fairly typical, people continue to get the impression that they are not taken seriously by the staff.

Anthropologists, particularly applied anthropologists, have discussed the problematic interactions between people and agencies that intend to foster development and improve health (e.g., Anglin 2002; Chernela 2005; Schensul 1999). Critical medical anthropologists note the imposition of "externally generated 'solutions' to externally determined health problems" and call instead for collaboration "with struggling communities and groups in responding to their felt needs" (Singer 1995:99). There is an urgent need for fostering trust and dialogue between health workers and communities (Pfeiffer 2004:96). The emphasis on improving interaction sounds simple, and my observations confirm that active listening—giving time and attention to people's words—is crucial to their acceptance of the medical advice and services of AIDS agencies. That I often witnessed agency staff failing to take this issue seriously motivated me to provide this information.

There are also positive examples from which we can learn (e.g., Romero-Daza 2005). In my observation, these are usually small-scale agencies with humble budgets and infrastructure but with people who take their time to sit down with people, discuss the various facets of the AIDS epidemic—including sorcery and conspiracy—and then try to develop local responses to the epidemic. They are successful in connecting the distinct cognitive worlds and in moving forward. They take seriously what Green (2003:330) advised those working in the field of AIDS awareness and prevention to do, namely, to "arrive with a sense of humility and a willingness to learn from our hosts, rather than simply with a determination to teach them, show them the error of their ways, and transfer technology."

I met representatives of another AIDS agency during my fieldwork. They trained groups of volunteers who provided home-based care for people suffering from full-blown AIDS. Their local headquarters were in one of the townships, in a garage adapted as offices. Whenever I visited their modestly equipped offices, I met people from the township talking without inhibition with the representatives of the agency. The agency's representatives were part of their social world and the offices were in a setting familiar to them. People expressed their trust in this agency, but distrust in some other agencies. People from the township came to request that members of the agency train them in home-based care. The agency's instructors went to visit the volunteers and stayed with them for a weekend or several days. When the place was far away from where the instructors lived, they stayed with members of the newly formed group. When they met, the instructors often just listened to the questions of the group and provided simple, practical answers when necessary. However, most times, people found the answers themselves during the discussions.

The strength of this AIDS agency is that it builds on local interests and the perceived needs of people. Instruction is flexible and geared to what people want to learn and to do. The agency's representatives hold workshops from time to time so that groups can share their experiences, find answers to their questions, and report on their efforts. During the workshops, sorcery and conspiracy suspicions regarding the origin of the AIDS epidemic are not taboo. The agency's representatives also provide modest remuneration for the travel expenses of the home-based caregivers; hand out some humble medical and other material support for the families of people suffering from full-blown AIDS; distribute vouchers for sick individuals who cannot afford going to the local clinic; and help them with communicating with the social welfare bureaucracy.

What can we learn from this rather long excursion into the realities of AIDS awareness, prevention, and care? I argue that, in order to inform people about the epidemic, to prevent new HIV infections, and to improve the care of those infected with the virus and those suffering from full-blown AIDS, we need to know and respond to the needs and views of the people. We have seen that many AIDS agencies are not taken seriously, thus compromising the success of their programs. Sorcery beliefs and conspiracy suspicions particularly represent a gap between the people's and the healthcare providers' concerns with HIV/AIDS, which needs to be addressed.

Three concerns that people express through a reference to sorcery and conspiracy seem to have a wide distribution across cultures. First, I observed that healthcare providers focused on the sexual, sanguinal, and perinatal transmission of HIV. I learned in interviews and in everyday contacts with Zimbabweans that they wanted information about the origin of AIDS, especially possible causes that explain the epidemic from a wider point of view. When they do not receive this information, they accept the information spread through the conspiracy theories locally, nationally, and worldwide. These theories have arisen from people's readings of the troubled history and prevailing conditions of the AIDS epidemic and rest in a societal, economic, and political context. They address issues of global economics and politics that are not simply products of paranoia but to some degree correct observations about how the world works.

Lacking satisfactory information, and with a history of neglect by the world's powers, Zimbabweans, like many in the developing world, commonly imagine that a cure for AIDS is available but is intentionally being withheld from them. Such suspicions color the whole problem of providing affordable ARV drugs in the developing world. Thus, some conspiracy theories can be seen as symbolic expressions of social, political, and economic problems across the world. Anthropologists have frequently interpreted sorcery in that way (e.g., Comaroff and Comaroff 1993, 1998). My observations corroborate such interpretations for certain conspiracy theories as well. Successful AIDS awareness, prevention, and care programs need to address such views. When AIDS agencies permit discussions on these popular themes and show their support for political efforts on both a national and global level to find solutions (e.g., to the affordable provision of ARV drugs), they will gain people's trust, which will improve the acceptance of their AIDS messages.

Second, I observed that prevention of new HIV infection was the main concern of the large AIDS organizations. But in interviews and everyday contacts I learned that people believing in sorcery and conspiracy are more concerned with finding the *origin* of the epidemic and, subsequently, a *cure*. During an interview, an old man summarized this common interest. He told me that, upon my return to the West, I should tell people that Zimbabweans are fed up with receiving condoms; instead, they need affordable medication for treating the symptoms of full-blown AIDS. He knew that in the West AIDS had become, through appropriate medication, more a chronic condition than a life-threatening disease. He was aware of the controversy over the prices of ARV drugs. He and others wanted affordable drugs for treatment—not condoms. Any discussion about the epidemic should connect to this fundamental concern of many individuals, and only then move on to other strategies to improve care. We need to listen to people, determine where they are in their thinking, and provide healthcare and education programs that move them forward. Such programs will offer pragmatic and realistic strategies that providers develop jointly with the people.

Third, I observed that many Zimbabweans attach morality to their AIDS beliefs. We have looked at this aspect of sorcery and conspiracy beliefs in the dog narrative, and in the suspicions that condoms are deliberately contaminated with HIV. I observed that the marketing of condoms neglected people's concern for their values.[1] In Zimbabwe a common poster shows young people "ready for action," furthering negative perceptions of condoms through association with promiscuous sexual behavior. Only once did I see a poster showing a middle-aged couple with children that promoted the use of condoms among couples where one of the spouses is HIV-positive. Because marketing generally ignores morality when promoting the use of condoms, it has unintentionally become connected to promiscuity.

When people should protect themselves, this makes it more difficult for them to choose condoms. Social marketing of condoms also encourages the popular belief that condoms are deliberately contaminated with HIV. Recall the logic behind this belief: condoms are connected to promiscuous behavior; promiscuous behavior results in HIV-infection; thus condoms are the cause of HIV-infection. I have observed the paradoxical situation in which programs meant to motivate young people to protect themselves from HIV-infection by using condoms actually contribute to the stigmatization of condoms—and thus potentially to new infections. To avoid such problems, marketers need to understand local morality and design materials that do not violate local standards.

In this regard, the ABC approach common in sub-Saharan Africa is ingenious (Green 2003; Green and Herling 2006): (A) if you are without a committed relationship, then abstain from sex; (B) if you are in a committed relationship, then be faithful to your partner; and (C) if you are not able to commit yourself to "A" or "B," then at least protect yourself and use a condom when you have sex. This approach takes into account that people ground their behavior in values, but realistically accepts that human weakness and shortcomings necessitate complementary strategies at times. Because ABC combines a value-based approach with a condom-based approach, it helps to remove some of the stigma from condoms. It gives the clear message that people who use condoms are good people acting responsibly.

Even the ABC approach can be scuttled by the lack of interaction between healthcare providers and their clients. This became evident when I attended a local church's workshop for young unmarried adults on the topic of preventing HIV-infection. The presenters aggressively attacked the ABC approach, reinterpreting it according to their own views. They said the "correct" ABC is the following: (A) abstain; (B) be faithful to your commitment to abstinence; and (C) if you cannot commit yourself to abstinence, then change—in other words, strengthen your commitment to abstinence.

Condoms were totally erased from this approach. The presenters emphasized the moral danger that condoms promote promiscuity and present a danger of infection. In a pseudoscientific explanation, the young people were told that HIV can quickly pass through the condoms. The presenters said because people feel safe using condoms during sexual intercourse, they increase their sexual activity, which then causes further HIV-infections. I talked to the presenters afterwards. They said they have no communication with agencies working in the field of AIDS prevention and awareness. Perhaps they did not want to work with AIDS agencies due to ideological differences; I did not observe any attempts by them or by AIDS staff to engage in dialogue.

Seeing human suffering on such a scale influenced my thinking. I observed the urgent need for cooperation—for all the agencies, groups, and individuals to try to understand and respect their different approaches and identify means of working together. The limited resources available makes it especially important to design effective strategies that allow people to choose the methods of prevention, and the types of care for those with AIDS, that meet their moral standards.

I am convinced that, underlying the various approaches and sometimes poorly carried out plans, AIDS workers in Zimbabwe share a concern for the victims. It is difficult, even painful, to observe the suffering and realize the limits of what can be done. I believe that underneath the superficial differences we share a common concern for human life that can bring us together. Beyond ideological differences and controversies all of us want to prevent new HIV-infections and to improve the condition of those suffering from full-blown AIDS.

Working together will help to bring forth the vision of the Zimbabwean lyricist Virginia Phiri (1998)[2]:

> We will never allow you [AIDS] to take us.
> We will fight you till our victory. . . .
> Herbalists, doctors, and churches are fighting you day and night.

Phiri's insight applies beyond the AIDS epidemic in Zimbabwe. Respectful communication and committed collaboration that take seriously the concerns of all involved will improve troubled relationships—the fertile ground for sorcery and conspiracy—and reduce mutual suspicions and blaming dynamics. A sincere effort to increase communication and collaboration among AIDS agencies, healthcare providers, and people who are suffering due to the AIDS epidemic could substantially transform prevention programs and bring compassion into the care of those suffering from AIDS.

Notes

1. For a concise summary of social marketing of condoms and a brilliant in-depth case study from Mozambique, see Pfeiffer 2004.
2. The Ndebele original was translated by Jabulani Mthombeni. Here is the original text: *Asisoze sikuvumele usithathe. Sizakulwisa size sinqobe. . . . Izinyanga, amadokotela kanye lamasonto, alwisana lawe emini lebusuku.*

Glossary

Abantu	plural of *umuntu*
Amagciwane	plural of *igciwane*
Amakhiwa	plural of *ikhiwa*
Apostle	member of one of the indigenous Apostle Churches
ARV	antiretroviral
Bulala	Ndebele verb for "to kill"
Cde.	Comrade
CIO	Central Intelligence Office
Dlisa	Ndebele verb for to "make to eat" or "feed"
DRC	Democratic Republic of Congo
Durawall	Precast concrete wall or fence
ESAP	Economic Structural Adjustment Policies
Gukurahundi	Fifth Brigade of the Zimbabwean army
HIV	human immunodeficiency virus
Igciwane	Ndebele term for "invisible insect," generally referring to a virus
Ikhiwa	derogatory Ndebele term for whites
Imikhoba	plural of *umkhoba*
Imithi	plural of *umuthi*
Imvukuzane	Ndebele term for cancer
Ingculaza	Variants of the Ndebele term for HIV/AIDS
Inhlonipho	Ndebele term for "respect" and/or "taboo"
Intokolosi	Variation of *intokolotshe*
Intokolotshe	Another Ndebele term for *undofa*
Inyanga	Ndebele term for "traditional healer"
Inyembezi	Ndebele term for "tears"
Isibungu	Ndebele term for a tiny insect or worm
Isidliso	Ndebele term for a form of sorcery poison added to food
Izibungu	plural of *isibungu*

Khiya	Ndebele term for "to lock"
MDC	Movement for Democratic Change
M.P.	Member of Parliament
n.d.	not dated
NGO	nongovernmental organization
Ngozi	sorcery practice that motivates spirits to revenge injustices
Prophet	Christian diviner and healer within indigenous churches
Runyoka	Shona term for *ulunyoka*
Sadza	Shona term referring to a stiff porridge made of grain meal
STD	sexually transmitted disease
TB	tuberculosis
Ulunyoka	Ndebele term for a particular sorcery poison as well as the ailment it causes in the lovers of married women
Umfundisi	Ndebele term for "minister of religion"
Umkhoba	Ndebele term for a sorcerer's familiar (similar to *undofa*)
Umkhuhlane	Ndebele term for "disease"
Umthakathi	Ndebele term for "sorcerer" or "witch"
Umuntu	Ndebele term for a human being, particularly of African descent
Umuthi	Ndebele term for "medicines" or "poisons"
UNAIDS	United Nations Program on HIV/AIDS
Undofa	Ndebele term for a particular sorcerer's familiar
Weltanschauung	Worldview
WHO	World Health Organization
ZANU-PF	Zimbabwe African National Union—Patriotic Front

Bibliography

Abalakina-Paap, Marina, and Walter G. Stephan
    1999   Beliefs in Conspiracies. *Political Psychology* 20(3):637–47.
Abramson, Paul R.
    1992   Sex, Lies, and Ethnographies. In *The Time of AIDS: Social Analysis, Theory, and Method.* G. Herdt and S. Lindenbaum, eds., pp. 101–123 Newbury Park: Sage.
Aggleton, Peter, Hilary Homans, Jan Mojsa, Stuart Watson, and Simon Watney
    1989   *AIDS: Scientific and Social Issues—A Resource for Health Educators.* Edinburgh: Churchill Livingstone.
Agresti, Alan, and Barbara Finlay
    1997   *Statistical Methods for the Social Sciences.* Upper Saddle River, NJ: Prentice Hall.
Aguirre Beltrán, Gonzalo
    1980   *Medicina y Magia: El Proceso de Aculturación en la Estructura Colonial.* Mexico City: Instituto Nacional Indigenista.
AIDS Control and Prevention Project
    1998   Report on KABP Impact Evaluation Survey on HIV/AIDS: National Railways of Zimbabwe (Draft), pp. 95. Harare.
Altman, Dennis
    1986   *AIDS in the Mind of America.* New York: Anchor Press.
Altman, Robert
    2001   *Gosford Park.* Hollywood: Universal Studio.
Anand, Raj, Alison Armstrong, Galabuzi Grace-Edward, Neve Alex, Rhea Whitehead, and Zimbabwe Reference Group.
    2004   *Zimbabwe Under Siege: A Canadian Civil Society Perspective.* No place of publication cited: Zimbabwe Reference Group.
Anderson, Jens A.
    2002   Sorcery in the Era of "Henry IV": Kinship, Mobility and Mortality in Buhera District, Zimbabwe. *Journal of the Royal Anthropological Institute* 8:425–449.
Anglin, Mary K.
    2002   Lessons from Appalachia in the 20th Century: Poverty, Power, and the "Grassroots." *American Anthropologist* 104(2):565–82.
Anonymous
    1986   AIDS: USA—Home-Made Evil, Not Imported from Africa. *Social Change and Development* (14):34–37.
    1987   AIDS Virus: Man-Made in the USA? *Border/lines* 9:7–8.

Anonymous (*continued*)

1990a	AIDS Help Line. *The Sunday News* (Bulawayo). October 14. P. 8.
1990b	Libyan Leader Muammar Gaddafi Blames US for AIDS. *The Sunday Mail* (Harare). July 22. P. 2.
1990c	Man on Remand for Bestiality. *The Herald* (Harare). May 18. P. 3.
1990d	*Dangerous Love.* Harare: Baobab Books.
1991a	AIDS and Runyoka: Are the Two Synonymous? *The Sunday Mail* (Harare). July 7. P. 9.
1991b	Chiefs Hit at Family Planning. *The Sunday News* (Bulawayo). May 19. P. 10.
1991c	Dog Brutalized. *The Chronicle* (Bulawayo). October 15. P. 6.
1991d	Dog Story Untrue. *The Herald* (Harare). October 10. P. 4.
1991e	Get the Dog's Side. Letter to the Editor. *The Chronicle* (Bulawayo). October 15. P. 3.
1991f	I Love. . . *The Herald* (Harare). September 13. P. 6.
1991g	Inhuman Sex Acts: Women Arrested. *The Sunday Mail* (Harare). September 29. P. 1
1991h	N'angas' Anti-AIDS Campaign Hits Snag. *The Chronicle* (Bulawayo). September 24. P. 11.
1994a	AIDS Created for Blacks—Doctor. *The Chronicle* (Bulawayo). August 2. P. 1–2.
1994b	Baboons Develop AIDS. *The Chronicle* (Bulawayo). October 29. P. 3.
1994c	McGown Got Anesthesia Technique from Journal. *The Herald* (Harare). August 2, pp. 1, 5.
1994d	Society Accused of Breaking Taboos. *The Herald* (Harare). March 9. P. 5.
1995	Faulty Condoms for Zimbabwe. *The Herald* (Harare). November 9. P. 7.
1996a	Disease Killed My Son—Nkomo Pleads for AIDS Cure. *The Sunday News* (Bulawayo). April 7. P. 1.
1996b	Men Held for Bestiality. *The Sunday News* (Bulawayo). September 1. P. 16.
1996c	My Son Died of AIDS—Nkomo Tells Mourners. *The Sunday Mail* (Harare). April 7, pp. 1, 4.
1997a	Patients Die During Experiments: Doctor Admits Illegal Tests. *The Chronicle* (Bulawayo). March 3, pp. 1, 5.
1997b	Witchcraft Act Criticized. *The Chronicle* (Bulawayo). March 1997. P. 7.
1998	A Thriller on How HIV Was Engineered. *The Chronicle* (Bulawayo). November 2. P. 8.
1999a	Racism Plays Role in AIDS Death Rate. *The Herald* (Harare). August 30. P. 2.
1999b	Shortage of Cemetery Space to Cope with AIDS Deaths. *The Herald* (Harare). November 4. P. 14.
1999c	South Africa Plays Down Faulty Condom Scare. *AIDS Weekly Plus* (January 11):10–11.
1999d	US Accused of Barring Access to AIDS Cure. *The Daily News* (Harare). April 13. P. 29.
2001a	Gaddafi Accuses United States of Creating AIDS. *The Daily News* (Harare). September 6. P. 4.
2001b	U.S. Created AIDS. *The Zimbabwe Independent* (Harare). April 12. P. 16.
2003a	AIDS Committees Lambasted. *The Chronicle* (Bulawayo). August 19. P. 2.

2003b	Bulawayo Families Surviving on One Meal a Day—Survey. *The Daily News* (Harare). July 25. P. 5.
2003c	Doctors Go on Strike. *The Chronicle* (Bulawayo). October 24. P. 2.
2003d	Free Treatment for HIV-Positive People. *The Chronicle* (Bulawayo). November 4. P. 7.
2003e	Government to Launch AIDS Prevention Program. *The Chronicle* (Bulawayo). July 31. P. 2.
2003f	Inflation Shoots Up to 445%. *The Chronicle* (Bulawayo). October 17. P. B 2.
2003g	Ministry of Health Advertises for 500 Posts. *The Chronicle* (Bulawayo). October 22. P. 2.
2004	Libyan Court Sentences Six to Death for Infecting Children with AIDS. *Health and Medicine Week*. May 24. P. 695. Electronic Document: http://lexis-nexis.com . Last Accessed: September 22, 2005.

Appel, W.
| 1977 | Idioms of Power in Southern Italy. *Dialectical Anthropology* 2:74–80. |

Ardener, Edwin
| 1970 | Witchcraft, Economics, and the Continuity of Belief. In *Witchcraft Confessions and Accusations*. Mary Douglas, ed., pp. 141–60. London: Tavistock Publications. |

Aristotle
| 1933 | *Metaphysics*: Books 1–14; *Oeconomica; Magna Moralia*. 2 Volumes. Translated by Tredennick, Hugh, and G. Cyril Armstrong. Cambridge: Harvard University Press. |
| 1934 | *Physics*. 2 Volumes. Translated by Wicksteed, P. H., and F. M. Cornford. Cambridge: Harvard University Press. |

Ashforth, Adam
1996	Of Secrecy and the Commonplace: Witchcraft and Power in Soweto. *Social Research* 63(4):1183–1234.
2000	*Madumo: A Man Bewitched.* Cape Town: David Philip Publishers.
2001a	AIDS, Witchcraft, and the Problem of Power in Post-Apartheid South Africa. In *Occasional Papers of the School of Social Sciences*, pp. 30. Cape Town.
2001b	On Living in a World with Witches: Everyday Epistemology and Spiritual Insecurity in a Modern African City (Soweto). In *Magical Interpretations, Material Realities: Modernity, Witchcraft and the Occult in Postcolonial Africa*. H.L. Moore and T. Sanders, eds., pp. 206–225. London: Routledge.
2002	An Epidemic of Witchcraft? The Implications of AIDS for the Post-Apartheid State. *African Studies* 61(1):121–43.
2005	*Witchcraft, Violence and Democracy in South Africa.* Chicago: University of Chicago Press.

Ashton, Hugh
| 1994 | Housing Policy and Practice: 1894–1994. In *Bulawayo: A Century of Development, 1894–1994*. M. Hamilton and M. Ndubiwa, eds., pp. 53–63. Harare: Argosy Press. |

Auslander, Mark
    1993   "Open the Wombs!": The Symbolic Politics of Modern Ngoni
                Witchfinding. In *Modernity and Its Malcontents: Ritual and Power in
                Postcolonial Africa*. J. Comaroff and J. Comaroff, eds., pp. 167–92.
                Chicago: University of Chicago Press.
Azevedo, Mario J.
    1989   Colonization, Settlement, and Urbanization in Southern Africa. In
                Preliminary Discussions on Problems of Urbanization in Southern Africa. A.
                Rother, ed., pp. 1–12. East Lansing: Michigan State University.
Bailey, Frederick George
    1994   *The Witch-Hunt, or the Triumph of Morality*. Ithaca: Cornell University
                Press.
Balikci, Asen
    1984   Netslik. *Handbook of North American Indians*. Volume 5, pp. 447–62.
Bassett, Mary Travis, and Marvellous Mhloyi
    1991   Women and AIDS in Zimbabwe: The Making of an Epidemic.
                International Journal of Health Services 21(1):143–56.
Bassett, Mary Travis, Leon Bijlmaker, and David Sanders
    1997   Professionalism, Patient Satisfaction, and Quality of Health Care:
                Experience During Zimbabwe's Structural Adjustment Programme.
                Social Science and Medicine 45(12):1845–52.
Beattie, John
    1963   Sorcery in Bunyoro. In *Witchcraft and Sorcery in East Africa*. J. Middleton
                and E.H. Winter, eds., pp. 27–55. New York: Frederick A. Praeger.
Beauvois, Jean-Leon, and Robert-Vincent Joule
    1998   Cognitive Dissonance Theory: A Radical View. *European Review of Social
                Psychology* 8:1–32.
Beck, Ann
    1985   Old and New Approaches to Medicine in Rhodesia and Zimbabwe.
                In *African Healing Strategies*. B.M. Du Toit and I.H. Abdalla, eds., pp.
                182–89. New York: Trado-Medic Books.
Beebe, J.
    1995   Basic Concepts and Techniques of Rapid Appraisal. *Human Organization*
                54:42–51.
Behar, Ruth
    1987   Sex and Sin, Witchcraft and the Devil in Late-Colonial Mexico. *American
                Ethnologist* 14(1):34–54.
Behringer, Wolfgang
    2004   *Witches and Witch-Hunts: A Global History*. Cambridge: Polity Press.
Beidelman, T. O.
    1963   Witchcraft in Ukaguru. In *Witchcraft and Sorcery in East Africa*. J.
                Middleton and E.H. Winter, eds., pp. 57–98. New York: Frederick A.
                Praeger.
    1970   Towards More Open Theoretical Interpretations. In *Witchcraft
                Confessions and Accusations*. Mary Douglas, ed., pp. 351–57. London:
                Tavistock.

Bennett, F. J.
1995   Qualitative and Quantitative Methods: In-depth or Rapid Assessment? *Social Science and Medicine* 40:1589–90.

Bennet, Richard M.
2003   *Conspiracies: Plots, Lies, and Cover-ups.* London: Virgin Books.

Berglund, Axel-Ivar
1976   *Zulu Thought-Patterns and Symbolism.* Studia Missionalia Upsaliensia: Volume XXII. Bloomington: Indiana University Press.
1989   Confessions of Guilt and Restoration of Health. Some Illustrative Zulu Examples. In *Culture, Experience, and Pluralism: Essays on African Ideas of Illness and Healing.* A. Jacobson-Widding and D. Westerlund, eds., pp. 109–124. Acta Universitatis Upsaliensis, Vol. 13. Uppsala: University of Uppsala.

Berlet, Chip
1997   Conspiracism. Electronic Document. http://www.publiceye.org/. Last Accessed: December 21, 2001.

Bernard, H. Russell
1996   Qualitative Data, Quantitative Analysis. *Cultural Anthropology Methods Journal* 8(1):9–11.
2002   *Research Methods in Anthropology: Qualitative and Quantitative Approaches.* Walnut Creek: AltaMira Press.

Bernstein, A. J., and C. A. J. van Rooyen
1994   Sociocultural Factors and Their Importance in Working with People with AIDS in South Africa. *Social Work/Maatskaplike Werk* 30(4):375–82.

Bird, Sheryl Thorburn, and Laura M. Bogart
2003   Birth Control, Conspiracy Beliefs, Perceived Discrimination, and Contraception among African Americans: An Exploratory Study. *Journal of Health Psychology* 8(2):263–76.
2005   Conspiracy Beliefs About HIV/AIDS and Birth Control Among African Americans: Implications for the Prevention of HIV, Other STIs, and Unintended Pregnancy. *Journal of Social Issues* 61(1):109–126.

Blackmore, Susan, and Richard Dawkins
1999   *The Meme Machine.* New York: Oxford University Press.

Bledsoe, Caroline
1990   The Politics of AIDS and Condoms for Stable Heterosexual Relations in Africa: Recent Evidence from the Local Print Media. In *Births and Power: Social Change and the Politics of Reproduction.* P.W. Handwerker, ed., pp. 197–222. Boulder, CO: Westview Press.

Bloomhill, Greta
1962   *Witchcraft in Africa.* Cape Town: Howard Timmins.

Blyth-Whiting, Beatrice
1950   *Paiute Sorcery.* Publications in Anthropology. Vol. 15. New York: Viking Fund.

Bogart, Laura M., and Sheryl Thorburn Bird
2003a   Exploring the Relationship of Conspiracy Beliefs about HIV/AIDS to Sexual Behavior and Attitudes among African American Adults. *Journal of the National Medical Association* 95(11):1057–65.

Bogart, Laura M., and Sheryl Thorburn Bird (continued)
2003b   Conspiracy Beliefs About HIV/AIDS to Sexual Behaviors and Attitudes among African-American Adults. *Journal of the National Medical Association.* 95(11):1057–65.
2005   Are HIV/AIDS Conspiracy Beliefs a Barrier to HIV Prevention Among African Americans? *Journal of Acquired Immune Deficiency Syndromes* 38:213–18.

Bogucka, Teresa
2001   Verschwörungstheorien in Polen: Reminiszenzen und Reflexionen. In *Verschwörungstheorien: Anthropologische Konstanten Historische Varianten.* U. Caumanns and M. Niendorf, eds., pp. 125–36. Osnabrück: Fibre.

Bond, George Clement
2001a   Ancestors and Witches: Explanations and the Ideology of Individual Power in Northern Zambia. In *Witchcraft Dialogues: Anthropological and Philosophical Exchanges.* G.C. Bond and Diane M. Ciekawy, eds., pp. 131–57. Athens, OH: Ohio University Center for International Studies.

Bond, George Clement, and Diane M. Ciekawy
2001   Contested Domains in the Dialogues of "Witchcraft." In *Witchcraft Dialogues: Anthropological and Philosophical Exchanges.* G.C. Bond and D.M. Ciekawy, eds., pp. 1–38. Athens, OH: Ohio University Center for International Studies.

Bond, Patrick
2001b   Radical Rhetoric and the Working Class During Zimbabwean Nationalism's Dying Days. In *Striking Back: The Labor Movement and the Post-Colonial State in Zimbabwe 1980–2000.* B. Raftopoulos and L. Sachikonye, eds., pp. 25–52. Harare: Weaver Press.

Bonner, C. A.
1950   *Studies in Magical Amulets, Chiefly Graeco-Egyptian.* Ann Arbor: University of Michigan Press.

Bourdillon, Michael F. C.
1976   *The Shona Peoples: An Ethnography of the Contemporary Shona, with a Special Reference to Their Religion.* Gweru, Zimbabwe: Mambo Press.
1993   *Where Are the Ancestors? Changing Culture in Zimbabwe.* Harare: University of Zimbabwe Publications.

Bowden, Ross
1987   Sorcery, Illness and Social Control in Kwoma Society. In *Sorcery and Witch in Melanesia.* Stephen, Michelle, ed., pp. 183–208. New Brunswick: Rutgers University Press.

Brain, James L.
1975   Witchcraft in Africa: A Hardy Perennial. In *Colonialism and Change: Essays Presented to Lucy Mair.* M. Owusu, ed., pp. 179–201. The Hague: Mouton.

Brain, R.
1970   Child-Witches. In *Witchcraft Confessions and Accusations,* Mary Douglas, ed., pp.161–83. London: Tavistock.

Brandt, Allan M.
  1988   AIDS and Metaphor: Toward the Social Meaning of Epidemic Disease.
            Social Research 55(3):413–32.
Bratich, Jack
  2002   Injections and Truth Serums: AIDS Conspiracy Theories and the Politics
            of Articulation. In *The Politics of Paranoia in Postwar America.* P. Knight,
            ed., pp. 133–56. New York: New York University Press.
Brettell, Caroline B.
  1998   Fieldwork in the Archives: Methods and Sources in Historical
            Anthropology. In *Handbook of Methods in Cultural Anthropology.* H.R.
            Bernard, ed., pp. 513–46. Walnut Creek: AltaMira Press.
Brickhill, Jeremy
  1992   Zimbabwe's Poisoned Legacy: Secret War in Southern Africa. *Covert
            Action* 43:4–59.
Briggs, Robin
  1996a   "Many Reasons Why": Witchcraft and the Problem of Multiple
            Explanation. In *Witchcraft in Early Modern Europe.* Barry, Jonathan;
            Marianne Hester and Gareth Roberts, eds., pp. 49–63. Cambridge:
            Cambridge University Press.
  1996b   *Witches and Neighbors: The Social and Cultural Context of European
            Witchcraft.* New York: Viking Penguin Books.
Brunvand, Jan Harold
  1981   *The Vanishing Hitchhiker: American Urban Legends and Their Meanings.*
            New York: W. W. Norton.
Buckley, Sandra
  1997   The Foreign Devil Returns: Packaging Sexual Practice and Risk in
            Contemporary Japan. In *Sites of Desire, Economies of Pleasure: Sexualities
            in Asia and the Pacific.* Lenore Manderson and Margaret Jolly, eds., pp.
            262-292. Chicago: University of Chicago Press.
Bullock, Charles
  1950   *The Mashona and the Matabele.* Cape Town: Juta & Co.
Bürger, Christine
  1999   *AIDS in Simbabwe: Armut oder Tradition als Ursache der Verbreitung.*
            Studien zur Afrikanischen Geschichte: Volume 24. Münster: LIT Verlag.
Butt, Leslie
  2005   "Lipstick Girls" and "Fallen Women": AIDS and Conspiratorial Thinking
            in Papua, Indonesia. *Cultural Anthropology* 20(3):412–42.
Caldwell, John, I. O. Orubuloye, and Pat Caldwell
  1992   Underreaction to AIDS in Sub-Saharan Africa. *Social Science and Medicine*
            34(11):1169–82.
Campbell, A. C.
  1918   Letter of the Native Commissioner from Belingwe to the Head Office
            in Salisbury. In *Folder A3 12/30/1 Vol. 1.* Harare: National Archives of
            Zimbabwe.

Cantwell, Alan
    1988   *The Doctors of Death: An Inquiry into the Origins of the AIDS Epidemic.* Los Angeles: Aries Rising Press.
    1993   *Queer Blood: The Secret AIDS Genocide Plot.* Los Angeles: Aries Rising Press.
    2002   Virus Wars: Does HIV Cause AIDS? In *Popular Paranoia: A Steamshovel Press Anthology.* Thomas, Kenn, ed., pp.83–89. Kempton: One Adventure Place.
Caprara, Andrea, Dedy Seri, Giulio C. de Gregorio, Alessandro Parenzi, Carlos M. Salazar, and Tape Goze
    1993   The Perception of AIDS in the Bete and Baoule of the Ivory Coast. *Social Science & Medicine* 36(9):1229–35.
Carneiro, Robert I.
    1977   Recent Observations on Shamanism and Witchcraft Among the Kuikuru Indians of Central Brazil. In *Anthropology and the Climate of Opinion. Annals of the New York Academy of Sciences.* Volume 293. Freed, Stanley A., ed., pp. 215–28.
Catholic Commission for Justice and Peace
    2000   *Crisis of Governance: A Report on Political Violence in Zimbabwe.* Volume 1. Harare.
Catholic Commission for Justice and Peace and Legal Resources Foundation
    1999   *Breaking the Silence: Building True Peace. A Report on the Disturbances in Matabeleland and the Midlands, 1980 to 1988: Summary Report.* Harare: Catholic Commission for Justice and Peace.
Central Statistical Office
    2001   *Education Statistics Report.* Harare: Government Printers.
Chamakuhwa, T.
    1991   The Animal Instinct in Man. *The Chronicle* (Bulawayo). October 26. P. 4.
Chari, Tendai Joseph
    2001   *The Impact of Mass Mediated HIV/AIDS Information on Behavior Change: The Case of University of Zimbabwe Students.* M. A. Media and Communication Studies. University of Zimbabwe.
Chavunduka, Gordon L.
    1982   *Witches, Witchcraft and the Law in Zimbabwe.* ZINATHA Occasional Paper: Volume 1. Harare: Matimba Printing Services.
    1986   ZINATHA: The Organization of Traditional Medicine in Zimbabwe. In *The Professionalization of African Medicine.* G.L. Chavunduka and M. Last, eds., pp. 29–49. Manchester: Manchester University Press.
    2001   *The Reality of Witchcraft.* African Legal Studies 2:163–69.
Cheater, Angela
    2001   *Human Rights and Zimbabwe's June 2000 Election.* Special Report: Volume 1. Harare: Zimbabwe Human Rights NGO Forum.
Chernela, Janet
    2005   The Politics of Mediation: Local-Global Interactions in the Central Amazon of Brazil. *American Anthropologist* 107(4):620–31.

Chikovore, J., and M. T. Mbizvo
1999   AIDS-related Knowledge and Sexual Behavior among Commercial Farm
        Residents in Zimbabwe. *Central African Journal of Medicine* 45(1):6–10.
Chikuhwa, Jacob
2004   *A Crisis of Governance: Zimbabwe.* New York: Algora Publishing.
Chikwanha, Annie, Tulani Sithole, and Michael Bratton
2004   The Power of Propaganda: Public Opinion in Zimbabwe, 2004.
        Afrobarometer Working Papers: Volume 42. Cape Town: IDASA POS.
Chimuchembere, Marizani
1992   AIDS Plot to Kill Blacks. *The Chronicle* (Bulawayo). September 20. P. 6.
Chirimuuta, Richard C., and Rosalind J. Chirimuuta
1989   *AIDS, Africa and Racism.* London: Free Association Books.
Chiroro, Patrick, Alexio Mashu, and William Muhwava
2002   *The Zimbabwean Male Psyche with Respect to Reproductive Health, HIV,
        AIDS, and Gender Issues.* Harare: University of Zimbabwe.
Chiweza, David
1997   *HIV and AIDS: The Last Stand: The Total Strategy for the Annihilation of
        HIV and AIDS in Zimbabwe and the Rest of the World.* Harare: Able City.
Chowning, Ann
1987   Sorcery and the Social Order in Kove. In *Sorcerer and Witch in Melanesia.*
        Stephen, Michelle, ed., pp. 149–82. New Brunswick: Rutgers University Press.
Chuma, Emmanuel
2003   Healer's Death Sends Shivers Down Spines: Many Errant Husbands
        Could Have Been Locked. Concerned Clients Jam Switchboard. *The
        Chronicle* (Bulawayo). August 16. P. 1.
Civic, Diane, and David Wilson
1996   Dry Sex in Zimbabwe and Implications for Condom Use. *Social Science
        and Medicine* 42(1):91–98.
Cirac Estopañán, Sebastián
1942   *Los Procesos de Hechicerias en la Inquisición de Castilla la Nueva*
        (Tribunales de Toledo y Cuenca). Madrid: CS/C.
Clark, P. A.
1998   A Legacy of Mistrust: African-Americans, the Medical Profession, and
        AIDS. *Linacre Quarterly* 87:66–88.
Cline, Rebecca, and Nelya J McKenzie
2000a   Dilemmas of Disclosure in the Age of HIV/AIDS: Balancing Privacy and
        Protection in the Health Care Context. In *Balancing the Secrets of Private
        Disclosures.* S. Petronio, ed., pp. 71–82. Mahwah: Erlbaum.
2000b   Interpersonal Roulette and HIV/AIDS Disability: Stigma and Social
        Support in Tension. In *Handbook of Communication and People with
        Disability.* D.O. Braithwaite and T. Thompson, eds., pp. 467–83.
        Mahwah: Erlbaum.
Coleman, Jane Dexter
1976   *The Social Expression of Paranoia: An Investigation of Some Situational
        Determinants of the Belief in Conspiracy.* Ph.D. Political Science. Columbia
        University.

Comaroff, Jean, and John Comaroff
    1993   Introduction. In *Modernity and Its Malcontents: Ritual and Power in Postcolonial Africa*. J. Comaroff and J. Comaroff, eds., pp. xi–xxxvii. Chicago: University of Chicago Press.
    1998   Occult Economies and the Violence of Abstraction: Notes from the South African Postcolony. *American Ethnologist* 26(2):279–303.

Comaroff, John, and Jean Comaroff
    1992   *Ethnography and the Historical Imagination*. Boulder: Westview Press.

Conco, W. Z.
    1979   The African Bantu Traditional Practice of Medicine: Some Preliminary Observations. In *African Therapeutic Systems*. Z.A. Ademuwagun, J. Ayoade, I.E. Harrison, and D.M. Warren, eds., pp. 58–80. Waltham: Crossroads Press.

Connelly, Nancy Diane
    1983   *Temporary Middlemen: Hindu and Moslem Asians in Bulawayo*. Ph.D. Dissertation. Anthropology. Southern Methodist University.

Coombe, Rosemary J.
    1997   The Demonic Place of the "Not There": Trademark Rumors in the Postindustrial Imaginary. In *Culture, Power and Place: Explorations in Critical Anthropology*. Gupta, Akhil and James Ferguson. Durham: Duke University Press.

Crane, Julia G., and Michael V. Angrosino
    1992   *Field Projects in Anthropology: A Student Handbook*. Prospect Heights: Waveland.

Crawford, J. R.
    1967   *Witchcraft and Sorcery in Rhodesia*. London: Oxford University Press.

Cress-Welsing, Frances
    1991   *The Isis Papers: The Keys to the Colors*. Chicago: Third World Press.

Crisis in Zimbabwe Coalition
    2003   Defiance versus Repression: Critical Reflections on the "Final Push", June 2–6, 2003. Harare: Crisis in Zimbabwe Coalition.

Crocker, Jennifer, Riia Luhtanen, Stephanie Broadnax, and Bruce Evan Blaine
    1999   Belief in U.S. Government Conspiracies Against Blacks Among Black and White College Students: Powerlessness or System Blame? *Personality and Social Psychology Bulletin* 25(8):941–53.

Darling, J. Andrew
    1999   Mass Inhumation and the Execution of Witches in the American Southwest. *American Anthropologist* 100(3):732–52.

Dashwood, Hevina
    2000   *Zimbabwe: The Political Economy of Transformation*. Toronto: University of Toronto Press.

Davis, D. G.
    1969   *The Slave Power Conspiracy and the Paranoid Style*. Baton Rouge: Louisiana State University Press.

de Blécourt, Willem
    1999   The Witch, her Victim, the Unwitcher and the Researcher: The Continued Existence of Traditional Witchcraft. In *Witchcraft and Magic*

in Europe: The Twentieth Century. Ankarloo, Bengt and Stuart Clark, eds., pp. 141–219. Philadelphia: University of Pennsylvania Press.

de Mello e Souza, Laura
    2003   *The Devil and the Land of the Holy Cross: Witchcraft, Slaves, and Popular Religion in Colonial Brazil.* Austin: University of Texas Press.

de Munck, Victor C.
    1998   Participant Observation: A Thick Description of Conflict in a Sri Lankan Village. In *Using Methods in the Field: A Practical Introduction and Casebook.* E.J. Sobo and V. C. de Munck, eds., pp. 39–54. Walnut Creek, CA: AltaMira Press.

de Walt, Kathleen M., Billie R. DeWalt, and Coral B. Wayland
    1998   Participant Observation. In *Handbook of Methods in Cultural Anthropology.* H.R. Bernard, ed., pp. 259–99. Walnut Creek: AltaMira Press.

Denzin, Norman
    1978   The Logic of Naturalistic Inquiry. In *Sociological Methods: A Sourcebook.* N. Denzin, ed., pp. 6–28. New York: McGraw-Hill.

DeParle, Jason
    1990   Talk of Government Being Out to Get Blacks Falls on More Attentive Ears. *The New York Times,* October 29:B7.

de Rosny, Eric
    1985   *Healers in the Night.* New York: Orbis Books.

Devisch, René
    2001   Sorcery Forces of Life and Death among the Yaka of Congo. In *Witchcraft Dialogues: Anthropological and Philosophical Exchanges.* G.C. Bond and D.M. Ciekawy, eds., pp. 101–130. Athens, OH: Ohio University Center of International Studies.

Dhliwayo, Rogers
    2001   The Impact of Public Expenditure Management under ESAP on Basic Social Services, Health and Education, pp. 30. Harare.

Dilger, Hansjörg
    1999   "*Besser der Vorhang im Haus als die Fahne im Wind*": Geld, AIDS, und Moral im ländlichen Tanzania. Spektrum: Volume 62. Hamburg: LIT Verlag.

Dillon-Malone, Clive
    1988   Mutumwa Nchimi Healers and Wizardry Beliefs in Zambia. *Social Science & Medicine* 26(11):1159–72.

Dlodlo, Riitta
    2002   City of Bulawayo: 2001 Annual Report of the Director of Health Services, pp. 50. Bulawayo.
    2003   City of Bulawayo: 2002 Annual Report of the Director of Health Services, pp. 54. Bulawayo.

Doka, Kenneth
    1997   *AIDS, Fear and Society: Challenging the Dreaded Disease.* Washington, DC: Taylor & Francis.

Dongozi, Foster
    2003   Vendors Making a Killing at the Cemetery. *The Daily News* (Harare). April 22, pp. 16–17.

Douglas, Mary

    1966   *Purity and Danger: An Analysis of the Concepts of Pollution and Taboo.*
London: Routledge & Kegan Paul.

    1970   Introduction: Thirty Years after Witchcraft, Oracles and Magic. In
Witchcraft Confessions and Accusations. M. Douglas, ed., pp. xiii–xxxviii.
London: Tavistock Publications.

    1980   *Edward Evans-Pritchard. Modern Masters.* New York: Viking Press.

    1992   *Risk and Blame: Essays in Cultural Theory.* London: Routledge.

Drew, R. S., G. Foster, and J. Chimita

    1996   Cultural Practices Associated with Death in the North Nyanga District of
Zimbabwe and Their Impact on Widows and Orphans. *Journal of Social
Development in Africa* 11(1):79–86.

Drew, R. S., C. Makufa, and G. Foster

    1998   Strategies for Providing Care and Support to Children Orphaned by
AIDS. *AIDS Care* 10(Supplement 1):9–15.

Dube, Frank

    2003a   Men Should Change Behavior. *The Chronicle* (Bulawayo). May 27. P. 4.

Dube, G.

    2003b   Council Meeting Minutes. Bulawayo.

Dube, Kingsley Dinga

    1994   City Looks to the Zambezi for Survival and Prosperity. In *Bulawayo: A
Century of Development, 1894–1994.* M. Hamilton and M. Ndubiwa, eds.,
pp. 43–45. Harare: Argosy Press.

Dube, Mlandeli

    2000   Umkhosi Lo Umkhulu. In *Imisebe Yelanga.* M. Sitsha, J.R. Nyathi, T.J.C.
Nkomo, K.N. Mathe, J. Ngozo, M. Dube, N.S. Sigogo, B.D. Ndlovu, D.
Moyo, and N. Hlumbayo, eds., pp. 83–85. Harare: College Press.

Duesberg, Peter

    1987   Retroviruses as Carcinogens and Pathogens: Expectations and Realities.
Cancer Research 47:1199–1220.

    1996   *Inventing the AIDS Virus.* Washington, DC: Regnery.

Duh, Samuel V.

    1991   *Blacks and AIDS: Causes and Origin.* Sage Series on Race and Ethnic
Relations: Volume 3. Newbury Park: Sage Publications.

Durkheim, Émile

    1974   *Sociology and Philosophy.* New York: The Free Press.

du Toit, Brian M.

    1965   Medicine and Anthropology. *South African Journal of Science* 61(2): 55–60.

    1971   The Isangoma: An Adaptive Agent Among the Urban Zulu.
Anthropological Quarterly 44(2):51–65.

    1985   Religion, Ritual and Healing Among Urban Black South Africans. In
African Healing Strategies. B.M. du Toit and I.H. Abdalla, eds., pp. 151–
79. New York: Trado-Medic Books.

    2005   Healing and Medicine: Healing and Medicine in Africa. In *Encyclopedia
of Religion.* Volume 6. Second Edition. Lindsay Jones, ed., pp. 3816–21.
Detroit: Thomson Gale.

Duveen, Gerard
    2001a   Ideas and Their Development: A Dialogue between Serge Moscovici and Ivana Markova. In *Social Representations: Explorations in Social Psychology.* S. Moscovici, ed., pp. 224–86. New York: New York University Press.
    2001b   The Power of Ideas. In *Social Representations: Explorations in Social Psychology.* S. Moscovici, ed., pp. 1–18. New York: New York University Press.

Ellen, Roy
    1993   Introduction. In *Understanding Witchcraft and Sorcery in Southeast Asia.* Watson, C. W., and Roy Ellen, eds., pp. 1–25. Honolulu: University of Hawaii Press.

Ellert, H.
    1993   *The Rhodesian Front War: Counter-Insurgency and Guerilla Warfare, 1962–1980, 2nd Edition.* Gweru, Zimbabwe: Mambo Press.

Engelhard, Phillipe, Abib Samb, and Moussa Seck
    1988   Flying Saucers and the Monkey Virus. In *Blaming Others: Prejudice, Race, and Worldwide AIDS.* R. Sabatier and J. Tinker, eds., pp. 57–60. Washington: Panos Institute.

Epstein, A. L.
    1967   Urbanization and Social Change in Africa. *Current Anthropology* 8(4):275–95.
    1974   Introduction. In *Contention and Dispute: Aspects of Law and Social Control in Melanesia.* Epstein, A. L., ed., pp. 1–39. Canberra: Australian National University Press.

Estes, Leland L.
    1985   *The Role of Medicine and Medical Theories in the Rise and Fall of Witch Hunts in England.* Ph. D. Dissertation, Department of History, University of Chicago.

Evans-Pritchard, Edward Evans
    1929   The Morphology and Function of Magic. *American Anthropologist* 31(4):619–41.
    1931   Sorcery and the Native Opinion. *Africa* 4:22–55.
    1976a   Some Reminiscences and Reflections on Fieldwork. In *Witchcraft, Oracles, and Magic among the Azande.* E. E. Evans-Pritchard, ed., pp. 240–54. London: Oxford University Press.
    1976b   *Witchcraft, Oracles, and Magic among the Azande.* Oxford: Oxford University Press.

Eves, Richard
    2003   AIDS and Apocalypticism: Interpretations of the Epidemic from Papua New Guinea. *Culture, Health, and Sexuality* 5(3):249–64.

Farmer, Paul
    1988   Bad Blood, Spoiled Milk: Bodily Fluids as Moral Barometers in Rural Haiti. *American Ethnologist* 15(1):62–83.
    1992   *AIDS and Accusation: Haiti and the Geography of Blame. Comparative Studies of Health Systems and Medical Care.* Berkeley: University of California Press.
    1994   AIDS-Talk and the Constitution of Cultural Models. *Social Science & Medicine* 38(6):801–809.

Farmer, Paul (*continued*)
  1999   *Infections and Inequalities: The Modern Plagues.* Berkeley: University of
            California Press.
Favret-Saada, Jeanne
  1989   Unbewitching as Therapy. *American Ethnologist* 16(1):40–56.
Feldman, Douglas A.
  1990   *Culture and AIDS.* New York: Praeger.
Feldskov, Thomas, and Anne Mette Frederiksen
  2000   Survey on the Knowledge on HIV: Madala, Jongwe, Siyamuninga,
            and Nemadziva Villages, Gokwe North District, Midlands Province,
            Zimbabwe, pp. 41. Harare.
Fenster, Mark
  1999   *Conspiracy Theories: Secrecy and Power in American Culture.* Minneapolis:
            University of Minnesota Press.
Fernandez, James
  1986   *Persuasions and Performances: The Play of Tropes in Culture.* Bloomington:
            Indiana University Press.
Fernando, D.
  1993   *AIDS and Intravenous Drug Use: The Influence of Morality, Politics, Social
            Science, and Race in the Making of a Tragedy.* Westport: Praeger.
Festinger, Leon
  1957   *A Theory of Cognitive Dissonance.* Stanford: Stanford University Press.
Fine, Garry Alan
  1992   Introduction: Toward a Framework for Contemporary Legends. In
            Manufacturing Tales: Sex and Money in Contemporary Legends. Gary Alan
            Fine, ed., pp. 1–42. Knoxville: University of Tennessee Press.
Finerman, Ruthbeth, and Linda Bennett
  1995   Guilt, Blame, and Shame: Responsibility in Health and Sickness. *Social
            Science & Medicine* 40(1):1–3.
Fleisher, Mark S., and Jennifer A. Harrington
  1998   Freelisting: Management at a Women's Federal Prison Camp. In *Using
            Methods in the Field: A Practical Introduction and Casebook.* V. C. de Munck
            and E. J. Sobo, eds., pp. 69–84. Walnut Creek: AltaMira Press.
Forge, Anthony
  1970   Prestige, Influence, and Sorcery: A New Guinea Example. In *Witchcraft
            Confessions and Accusations.* Douglas, Mary, ed., pp. 257–75. London: Tavistock.
Forster, Peter Glover
  1998   Religion, Magic, Witchcraft, and AIDS in Malawi. *Anthropos* 93:537–45.
Forth, Gregory
  1993   Social and Symbolic Aspects of the Witch Among the Nage of Eastern
            Indonesia. In *Understanding Witchcraft and Sorcery in Southeast Asia.*
            Watson, C. W., and Roy Ellen, eds., pp. 99–122. Honolulu: University
            of Hawaii Press.
Foster, George M.
  1965   Peasant Society and the Image of Limited Good. *American Anthropologist*
            67(2):293–315.

1976   Disease Etiologies in Non-Western Medical Systems. *American Anthropologist* 78(4):773–82.

France, D.

1998   Challenging the Conventional Stance on AIDS. *The New York Times.* December 22. P. F6.

Freimuth, Vicki S., Sandra Crouse Quinn, Stephen B. Thomas, Galen Cole, Eric Zook, and Ted Duncan

2001   African Americans' Views on Research and the Tuskegee Syphilis Study. *Social Science & Medicine* 52:797–808.

Freyre, Gilberto

1966   *The Masters and the Slaves: A Study in the Development of Brazilian Civilization.* New York: Alfred A. Knopf.

Friedrich, Paul

1996   The Culture in Poetry and the Poetry in Culture. In *Culture/Contexture: Explorations in Anthropology and Literary Studies.* E. V. Daniel and J. M. Peck, eds., pp. 37–57. Berkeley: University of California Press.

Fry, G.

1975   *Night Riders in Black Folk History.* Knoxville: University of Tennessee Press.

Gadon, M., R. M. Chierici, and P Rios

2001   Afro-American Migrant Farmworkers: A Culture in Isolation. *AIDS Care* 13(6):789–801.

Galt, Anthony H.

1991   Magical Misfortune in Locorontondo. *American Ethnologist* 18(4):735–50.

Games, Dianna

2002   *The Zimbabwean Economy: How Has It Survived and How Will It Recover?* SAIIA Report: Volume 30. No place of publication cited: The South African Institute of International Affairs.

Gasch, H., Poulson, D. M. Fullilove, R. E., and M. T. Fullilove

1991   Shaping AIDS Education and Prevention Programs for African Americans Amidst Community Decline. *Journal of Negro Education* 60(1):85–96.

Geer, Ben

1998   *Something More Sinister.* Reading, UK: Access Marketing and Publishing.

Geisler, Wolff

1994   *AIDS, Origin, Spread and Healing.* Köln: Verlag Wolff Geisler.

Gelfand, Michael

1944   *Medical Problems in the Native of Southern Rhodesia.* NADA—The Rhodesia Ministry Internal Affairs Annual 21:33–38.

1967   *The African Witch: With Particular Reference to Witchcraft Beliefs and Practice among the Shona of Rhodesia.* Edinburgh: Livingstone.

1985   The Traditional Medical Practitioner in Zimbabwe: His Principles of Practice and Pharmacopoeia. Gweru, Zimbabwe: Mambo Press.

Gentilcore, David

1992   *From Bishop to Witch: The System of the Sacred in Early Modern Terra d'Otranto.* Manchester: Manchester University Press.

Geschiere, Peter
　　1997　　　The Modernity of Witchcraft: Politics and the Occult in Postcolonial Africa. Charlottesville: University Press of Virginia.
　　1998　　　Globalization and the Power of Indeterminate Meaning: Witchcraft and Spirit Cults in Africa and East Asia. Development and Change 29: 811–37.
Gijswijt-Hofstra, Marijke
　　1999　　　Witchcraft after the Witch-Trials. In Witchcraft and Magic in Europe: The Eighteenth and Nineteenth Centuries. Ankarloo, Bengt and Stuart Clark, eds., pp. 95–190. Philadelphia: University of Pennsylvania Press.
Gilbert, David
　　1996　　　Tracking the Real Genocide: AIDS, Conspiracy or Unnatural Disaster? Covert Action Quarterly (September 21):55–58.
　　1998　　　AIDS Conspiracy? Tracking Down the Real Genocide. Turning the Tide—L. A. Anti-Racism Newsletter 10(4):11–13.
Glass-Coffin, B.
　　1991　　　Discourse, Daño and Healing in North Coastal Peru. Medical Anthropology 13(1-2):33–55.
Glick, Leonard B.
　　1967　　　Medicine as an Ethnographic Category: The Gimi of the New Guinea Highlands. Ethnology 6:31–56.
Gluckman, Max
　　1965　　　The Ideas in Barotse Jurisprudence. New Haven: Yale University Press.
　　1966　　　Custom and Conflict in Africa. Oxford: Blackwell Publishers.
　　1970　　　The Logic of African Science and Witchcraft. In Witchcraft and Sorcery: Selected Readings. M. Marwick, ed., pp. 321–31. Harmondsworth: Penguin Books.
Goertzel, Ted
　　1994　　　Belief in Conspiracy Theories. Political Psychology 15(4):731–42.
Goffman, Erving
　　1959　　　The Presentation of Self in Everyday Life. Garden City: Doubleday.
　　1963　　　Stigma: Notes on the Management of Spoiled Identity. Englewood Cliffs, NJ: Prentice-Hall Inc.
Goldberg, Robert Alan
　　2001　　　Enemies Within: The Culture of Conspiracy in Modern America. New Haven: Yale University Press.
Goldstein, Diane E.
　　2004　　　Once Upon a Virus: AIDS Legends and Vernacular Risk Perception. Logan: Utah State University Press.
Golomb, Louis
　　1985　　　An Anthropology of Curing in Multiethnic Thailand. Urbana: University of Illinois Press.
　　1993　　　The Relativity of Magical Malevolence in Urban Thailand. In Understanding Witchcraft and Sorcery in Southeast Asia. Watson, C. W., and Roy Ellen, eds., pp. 27–45. Honolulu: University of Hawaii Press.
Gonzales, Nancie L. Solien
　　1989　　　Belize: Black Caribs. In Witchcraft and Sorcery of the American Native

Peoples. Walker, Deward E., ed., pp. 279–93. Moscow: University of Idaho Press.

Good, Byron J.
1994   *Medicine, Rationality and Experience. An Anthropological Perspective.* Cambridge: Cambridge University Press.

Good, Charles M.
1987   *Ethnomedical Systems in Africa.* New York: Guilford.

Goodwin, Robin and Alexandra Kozlova, Anna Kwiatkowska, Lan Anh Nguyen Luu, George Nizharadze, Anu Realo, Ahto Külvet, Andu Rämmer
2003   Social Representations of HIV/AIDS in Central and Eastern Europe. *Social Science and Medicine* 56:1373–84.

Gordon, Richard
1999   Imagining Greek and Roman Magic. In *Witchcraft and Magic in Europe: Ancient Greece and Rome.* Ankarloo, Bengt and Stuart Clark, eds., pp. 159–276. Philadelphia: University of Pennsylvania Press.

Government Town Planning Office (Bulawayo)
1951   *Town and Country Planning with Special Reference to Bulawayo Peri-Urban Areas.* Bulawayo: The Rhodesia Printing & Publishing Co.

Grant, Miriam, and Andrew Palmiere
2003   When Tea Is a Luxury: The Economic Impact of HIV/AIDS in Bulawayo, Zimbabwe. *African Studies* 62(2):213–41.

Graubard, Mark
1984   *Witchcraft and the Nature of Man.* Lanham: University Press of America.

Graumann, Carl F.
1987   Conspiracy: History and Social Psychology: A Synopsis. In *Changing Conceptions of Conspiracy.* C. F. Graumann and S. Moscovici, eds., pp. 245–51. Springer Series in Social Psychology. New York: Springer-Verlag.

Graumann, Carl F., and Serge Moscovici
1987   Preface. In *Changing Conceptions of Conspiracy.* C. F. Graumann and S. Moscovici, eds. Springer Series in Social Psychology. New York: Springer-Verlag.

Gray, Fred D.
1998   *The Tuskegee Syphilis Study.* Montgomery: New South Books.

Green, Edward C.
1999   *Indigenous Theories of Contagious Disease.* Walnut Creek: AltaMira Press.
2003   *Rethinking AIDS Prevention: Learning from Successes in Developing Countries.* Westport: Praeger.

Green, Edward C. and A. Herling
2006   *A Primer on the ABC Approach to HIV Prevention: Common Questions and Answers about the ABC Approach to HIV Prevention.* Washington: Christian Connections for International Health.

Greenspan, David W, and Christopher Wilson
1989   Knowledge about AIDS and Self-Reported Behavior Among Zimbabwean Secondary School Pupils. *Social Science and Medicine* 28:957–61.

Gregson, Simon, Geoffrey P. Garnett, Constance A. Nyamukapa, Timothy B. Hallett, James J. C. Lewis, Peter R. Mason, Stephen K. Chandiwana, and Roy M. Anderson
   2006   HIV Decline Associated with Behavior Change in Eastern Zimbabwe. *Science* 311(3 February 2005): 664–66.
Gregson, Simon, Tom Zhuwau, Roy M. Anderson, and Steven K. Chandiwana
   1998   Is There Evidence for Behavior Change in Response to AIDS in Rural Zimbabwe? *Social Science and Medicine* 46(3):321–30.
Greunke, Gudrun
   2001   The Cooking Oil Conspiracy. *The Ecologist* 31(6):48–49.
Groh, Dieter
   1987   The Temptation of Conspiracy Theory, Or: Why Do Bad Things Happen to Good People? Part 1: Preliminary Draft of a Theory of Conspiracy Theories. In *Changing Conceptions of Conspiracy*. C. F. Graumann and S. Moscovici, eds., pp. 1–13. Springer Series in Social Psychology. New York: Springer-Verlag.
   2001   Verschwörungstheorien Revisited. In *Verschwörungstheorien: Anthropologische Konstanten Historische Varianten*. U. Caumanns and M. Niendorf, eds., pp. 187–96. Osnabrück: Fibre.
Grundlingh, Louis
   1999   HIV/AIDS in South Africa: A Case of Failed Responses Because of Stigmatization, Discrimination, and Morality; 1983–1994. *New Contree* 46(November):55–81.
Guinan, Mary E.
   1993   Black Communities' Belief in "AIDS as Genocide": A Barrier to Overcome for HIV Prevention. *Annals of Epidemiology* 3(2):193–95.
Gulbrandsen, Ørnulf
   2002   The Discourse of "Ritual Murder": Popular Reaction to Political Leaders in Botswana. In *Beyond Rationalism: Rethinking Magic, Witchcraft and Sorcery*. B. Kapferer, ed., pp. 215–33. New York: Berghahn Books.
Gumbo, Justine
   1991   What a Disgrace! Letter to the Editor. *The Chronicle* (Bulawayo). October 12, p. 5.
Gusfield, Joseph
   1981   *The Culture of Public Problems: Drinking-Driving and the Symbolic Order.* Chicago: Chicago University Press.
Gussman, B. W.
   1952   *African Life in an Urban Area: A Study of the African Population of Bulawayo.* 1. Bulawayo: The Federation of African Welfare Societies in Southern Rhodesia.
Gusterson, Hugh
   2004   How Far Have We Traveled? Magic, Science, and Religion Revisited. *Anthropology News* 45(8):7, 11.
Hallen, B., and J. O. Sodipo
   1986   *Knowledge, Belief and Witchcraft.* London: Ethnographica.
Hammond-Tooke, David
   1993   *The Roots of Black South Africa.* Johannesburg: Jonathan Ball Publishers.

Handwerker, Penn

1998   Consensus Analysis: Sampling Frames for Valid, Generalizable Research Findings. In *Using Methods in the Field: A Practical Introduction and Casebook*. V.C. de Munck and E.J. Sobo, eds., pp. 165–78. Walnut Creek: AltaMira Press.

2001   *Quick Ethnography*. Walnut Creek: AltaMira Press.

Hannerz, Ulf

1987   The World of Creolization. *Africa* 57(4):546–59.

Hansen, Kristian, Glyn Chapman, Inam Chitsike, Ossy Kasilo, and Gabriel Mwaluko

2000   The Costs of HIV/AIDS Care at Government Hospitals in Zimbabwe. *Health Policy and Planning* 15(4):432–40.

Harmon-Jones, Eddie

2000   A Cognitive Dissonance Theory Perspective on the Role of Emotions in the Maintenance and Change of Beliefs and Attitudes. In *Emotions and Beliefs: How Feelings Influence Thoughts*. N. Frijda, A. Manstead, and S. Bem, eds., pp. 185–211. Cambridge: Cambridge University Press.

Harper, Douglas

1988   Visual Sociology: Expanding Sociological Vision. *American Sociologist* 19(Spring):54–70.

Harris, Marvin

1975   *Cows, Pigs, Wars and Witches: The Riddles of Culture*. New York: Vintage Books.

1976   History and Significance of the Emic/Etic Distinction. *Annual Review of Anthropology* 5:329–50.

Harter, Jennifer

1998   *The Relationship Between Blame Attributions, Perceived Benefits and Psychological Adaptation in Adults with HIV/AIDS*. Ph.D. Dissertation. Psychology. Fordham University.

Harwood, Alan

1970   *Witchcraft: Sorcery and Social Categories among the Safwa*. London: Oxford University Press.

Hasler, Richard

1989   Historical Development and Problems of Urbanization in Southern Africa with a Focus on Zimbabwe. In *Preliminary Discussions on Problems of Urbanization in Southern Africa*. A. Rother, ed., pp. 13–22. East Lansing: Michigan State University.

Hastrup, Kirsten

1990   *Island of Anthropology: Studies in Past and Present Iceland*. Odense: University Press.

Hawkins, Denise B.

2005   On the Frontline of the HIV/AIDS Epidemic. *Black Issues in Higher Education* 22(3):24–29.

Hellinger, D.

2003   Paranoia, Conspiracy, and Hegemony in American Politics. In *Transparency and Conspiracy: Ethnographies of Suspicion in the New World Order*. Harry G. West and Todd Sanders, eds., pp. 204–232. Durham: Duke University Press.

Hendershot, Cyndy
    1999   *Paranoia, the Bomb, and 1950s Science Fiction Films.* Bowling Green: Bowling Green State University Popular Press.

Herdt, Gilbert, and Robert Stoller
    1990   *Intimate Communications: Erotics and the Study of Culture.* New York: Columbia University Press.

Herek, Gregory M., and John P. Capitanio
    1994   Conspiracies, Contagion, and Compassion: Trust and Public Reactions to AIDS. *AIDS Education and Prevention* 6(4):365–75.

Herek, Gregory M. and E. K. Glunt
    1991   AIDS-Related Attitudes in the United States: A preliminary Conceptualization. *Journal of Sex Research* 28:99–123.

Herzfeld, Michael
    1981   Meaning and Morality: A Semiotic Approach to Evil Eye Accusations in a Greek Village. *American Ethnologist* 8:560–74.

Herzlich, Claudine
    1995   Modern Medicine and the Quest for Meaning: Illness as a Social Signifier. In *The Meaning of Illness: The Anthropology, History, and Sociology of Illness.* M. Auge and C. Herzlich, eds., pp. 151–74. Luxembourg: Harwood Academic Publishers.

Hewstone, Miles
    1989   *Causal Attribution: From Cognitive Processes to Collective Beliefs.* Oxford: Basil Blackwell.

Hoebel, E. Adamson
    1952   Keresan Witchcraft. *American Anthropologist* 54(4):586–89.

Hofstadter, Richard
    1965   The Paranoid Style in American Politics. In *The Paranoid Style in American Politics and Other Essays.* R. Hofstadter, ed., pp. 3–40. Cambridge: Harvard University Press.

Honigmann, John J.
    1947   Witch-Fear in Post-Contact Kaska Society. *American Anthropologist* 49(2):222–43.

Hooper, E.
    1999   *The River: A Journey to the Source of HIV and AIDS.* New York: Little, Brown.

Horton, Leslie Ann
    1996   *"Eating Hearts": Witchcraft as Soul Murder. An Analysis of an Anti-Witch Youth Rebellion in Cameroon.* Ph.D. Dissertation. Anthropology. University of California.

Hove, Masotsha M.
    1985   *Confessions of a Wizard: A Critical Examination of the Belief System of a People Based Mainly on Personal Experience.* Gweru (Zimbabwe): Mambo Press.

Hunter-Wilson, Monica
    1970   Witch-Beliefs and Social Structure. In *Witchcraft and Sorcery: Selected Readings.* M. Marwick, ed., pp. 252–63. Harmondsworth: Penguin Books.

Hutchings, Anne, Alan Haxton-Scott, Gillian Lewis, and Anthony Cunningham
    1996   *Zulu Medicinal Plants: An Inventory.* Scottsville, South Africa: University of Natal Press.
Huygens, Pierre, Ellen Kajura, and Janet Seeley
    1996   Rethinking Methods for the Study of Sexual Behavior. *Social Science & Medicine* 42(2):221–31.
Huyssteyn, van Linda
    2002   The Influence of Culture in Zulu Language Development. In *Challenges for Anthropology in the "African Renaissance": A Southern African Contribution.* D. Le Beau and R.J. Gordon, eds., pp. 217–24. Windhoek: University of Namibia Press.
Ibarra, Peter R., and John I. Kitsuse
    1993   Vernacular Constituents of Moral Discourse: An Interactionist Proposal for the Study of Social Problems. In *Constructionist Controversies: Issues in Social Problems.* Miller, Gale, and James A. Holstein, eds., pp. 21–54. Hawthorne: Aldine de Gruyter.
Ingstad, Benedicte
    1989   Healer, Witch, Prophet or Modern Health Worker? The Changing Role of Ngaka Ya Setswana. In *Culture, Experience, and Pluralism: Essays on African Ideas of Illness and Healing.* A. Jacobson-Widding and D. Westerlund, eds., pp. 247–76. Acta Universitatis Upsaliensis, Vol. 13. Uppsala: University of Uppsala.
International Consortium of Investigative Journalists
    2002   *The Business of War: Making a Killing,* pp. 79. Place of publication not cited: The Center of Public Integrity.
International Crisis Group
    2003   *Zimbabwe: Danger and Opportunity.* Brussels: International Crisis Group.
Irwin, Kathleen, Jane Bertrand, Ndilu Mibandumba, Kashama Mbuyi, Chirezi Muremeri, Makolo Mukoka, Kamenga Munkolenkole, Nzila Nzilambi, Ngaly Bosenge, Robert Ryder, D Peterson, Elizabeth F Lee, Phyllis Wingo, K O'Reilly, and Kathy Rufo
    1991   Knowledge, Attitudes and Beliefs about HIV Infection and AIDS Among Healthy Factory Workers and Their Wives, Kinshasa, Zaire. *Social Science and Medicine* 32(8):917–30.
Jackson, Helen
    1988   *AIDS Action Now: Information, Prevention, and Support in Zimbabwe.* Harare: AIDS Counseling Trust.
    1999   A Note on National Policy and HIV/AIDS in Zimbabwe. In *AIDS and Development in Africa: A Social Science Perspective.* R. Kempe, ed., pp. 135–41. New York: Haworth Press.
    2002   *AIDS Africa: Continent in Crisis.* Harare: SAfAIDS.
Jackson, Helen, Russell Kerkhoven, Diane Lindsey, Gladys Mutangadura, and Fungayi Nhara
    1999   *HIV/AIDS in Southern Africa: The Threat to Development.* Harare: SAfAIDS.
Jackson, Helen, and Kate Mhambi
    1992   *AIDS Home Care: A Baseline Survey in Zimbabwe.* Research Series: Volume 3. Harare: School of Social Work.

Jackson, Helen, and Kate Mhambi (continued)
1994   Family Coping and AIDS in Zimbabwe: A Study. Research Unit Series:
            Volume 4. Harare: School of Social Work.
Jacques-Chaquin, Nicole
1987   Demoniac Conspiracy. In Changing Conceptions of Conspiracy. Graumann,
            Carl and Serge Moscovici, eds., pp. 71–85. New York: Springer.
Jameson, Frederic
1988   Cognitive Mapping. In Marxism and the Interpretation of Culture. C.
            Nelson and L. Grossberg, eds., pp. 347–60. Urbana: University of
            Illinois.
Jaworski, Rudolf
2001   Verschwörungstheorien aus psychologischer und aus historischer
            Sicht. In Verschwörungstheorien: Anthropologische Konstanten Historische
            Varianten. U. Caumanns and M. Niendorf, eds., pp. 11 30. Osnabrück:
            Fibre.
Jelmsa, Jennifer, Kristian Hansen, de Willy Weerdt, de Paul Cock, and Paul Kind
2003   How Do Zimbabweans Value Health States? Population Health Metrics
            1(11).
Joffe, Hélène
1996   AIDS Research and Prevention: A Social Representational Approach.
            British Journal of Medical Psychology 69:169–90.
1999   Risk and the "Other." Cambridge: Cambridge University Press.
Johwa, Wilson
2004   Health Zimbabwe: Provision of AIDS Drugs Fragmented. Electronic
            Source: http://ipsnews.net. Last Accessed: June 4, 2004.
Jones, James H.
1981   Bad Blood: The Tuskegee Syphilis Experiment. New York: The Free Press.
Joralemon, Donald and Douglas Sharon
1993   Sorcery and Shamanism: Curanderos and Clients in Northern Peru. Salt
            Lake City: University of Utah Press.
Jordan, Brigitte
1993   Birth in Four Cultures: A Cross-Cultural Investigation of Childbirth in
            Yucatan, Holland, Sweden, and the United States. Revised and Expanded
            by Robbie Davis-Floyd. Prospect Heights: Waveland.
Kaarsholm, Preben
1994   Si Ye Pambili—Which Way Forward? Urban Development, Culture, Politics
            in Bulawayo. Occasional Paper: Volume 146. Calcutta: Weaver Press.
Kaetzler, Joachim
2001   Magie und Strafrecht in Südafrika. Europäische Hochchulschriften:
            Volume 3218. Frankfurt am Main: Peter Lang.
Kagoro, Brian
2003   The Opposition and Civil Society. In Zimbabwe's Turmoil: Problems and
            Prospects. B. Kagoro, J. Makumbe, J. Robertson, P. Bond, E. Lahiff, and
            R. Cornwell, eds., pp. 4–16. Harare: Institute for Security Studies.
Kala, Violet
1994   Waste Not Your Tears. Harare: Baobab Books.

Kaler, Amy
    1998   A Threat to the Nation and a Threat to the Men: The Banning of Depo-Provera in Zimbabwe, 1981. *Journal of Southern African Studies* 24(2):347–76.
    2003   *Running After Pills: Politics, Gender, and Contraceptives in Colonial Zimbabwe. Social History of Africa*. Portsmouth: Heinemann.

Kapferer, Bruce
    1997   *The Feast of the Sorcerer: Practices of Consciousness and Power*. Chicago: University of Chicago Press.
    2002   Introduction: Outside All Reason: Magic, Sorcery, and Epistemology in Anthropology. In *Beyond Rationalism: Rethinking Magic, Witchcraft, and Sorcery*. B. Kapferer, ed., pp. 1–30. New York: Berghahn Books.

Kapferer, Jean-Noel
    1990   *Rumors: Uses, Interpretations, Images*. New Brunswick: Transaction.

Karim, Abdool
    1993   Traditional Healers and AIDS Prevention. *South African Medical Journal* 83(6):423–25.

Kasule, J., M. T. Mbizvo, V. Gupta, S. Fusakaniko, R. Mwateba, W. Mpanju-Shumbusho, S. H. Kinoti, and J. Padachy
    1997   Zimbabwean Teenagers' Knowledge of AIDS and Other Sexually Transmitted Diseases. *East African Medical Journal* 74(2):76–81.

Keeley, Brian L.
    1999   Of Conspiracy Theories. *Journal of Philosophy* 96(3):109–126.

Keller, Bonnie B.
    1978   Marriage and Medicine: Women's Search for Love and Luck. *African Social Research* 26:489–505.

Kelly, Michael
    1995   The Road to Paranoia. *The New Yorker*, June 19, pp. 60–75.

Kelly, Raymond C.
    1993   *Constructing Inequality: The Fabrication of a Hierarchy of Virtue Among the Etoro*. Ann Arbor: University of Michigan Press.

Kennedy, John
    1969   Psychosocial Dynamics of Witchcraft Systems. International *Journal of Social Psychiatry* 15(3):165–78.

Kiernan, Peter Miner
    1977   *Witchcraft, Sorcery, and Social Change in Africa: The Paradigm of Chewa Society*. M. A. African Studies. State University of New York.

Kilpatrick, Alan
    1997   *The Night Has a Naked Soul: Witchcraft and Sorcery among the Western Cherokee*. New York: Syracuse University Press.

Kimbrell, Andrew
    1993   Biotech Could Create "Super AIDS." *The Herald* (Harare). December 1. P. 6.

Kleinman, Arthur, L. Eisenberg, and B. Good
    1978   Culture, Illness, and Care: Clinical Lessons from Anthropologic and Cross-Cultural Research. *Annals of Internal Medicine* 88:251–58.

Kleinman, Arthur M.
1980   *Patients and Healers in the Context of Culture.* Berkeley: University of California Press.

Kleivan, Inge
1984   *West Greenland Before 1950.* Handbook of North American Indians. Volume 5, pp. 595–621.

Klonoff, Elizabeth A., and Hope Landrine
1999   Do Blacks Believe That HIV/AIDS Is a Government Conspiracy Against Them? *Preventive Medicine* 28:451–57.

Kluckhohn, Clyde
1944   *Navaho Witchcraft.* Boston: Beacon Press.

Knight, Francis Alfred
1994   Administrative History of Bulawayo. In *100 Years of Industry in Bulawayo: 1894–1994,* pp. 45–76. Bulawayo: Matabeleland Chamber of Industries.

Knight, Peter
2000   *Conspiracy Culture: From the Kennedy Assassination to the* X-Files. London: Routledge.

Knopf, Terry Ann
1975   *Rumors, Race, and Riots.* New Brunswick: Transaction Press.

Kramer, Roderick M.
1994   The Sinister Attribution Error: Paranoid Cognition and Collective Distrust in Organizations. *Motivation and Emotion* 18(2):199–230.

Krige, Eileen Jensen
1936   *The Social System of the Zulus.* Pietermaritzburg: Shuter and Shooter.

Krige, J. D.
1970   The Social Function of Witchcraft. In *Witchcraft and Sorcery: Selected Readings.* M. Marwick, ed., pp. 237–51. Harmondsworth: Penguin Books.

Kroeger, Karen A.
2003   AIDS Rumors, Imaginary Enemies, and the Body Politic in Indonesia. *American Ethnologist* 30(2):243–57.

Kruger, Steven F.
1996   *AIDS Narratives: Gender and Sexuality, Fiction and Science.* New York: Garland Publishing.

Kruglanski, Arie
1987   Blame-Placing Schemata and Attributional Research. In *Changing Conceptions of Conspiracy.* C. F. Graumann and S. Moscovici, eds., pp. 219–29. Springer Series in Social Psychology. New York: Springer-Verlag.

Lamphere, Louise
1971   The Navaho Cultural System: An Analysis of Concepts of Cooperation and Autonomy and Their Relation to Gossip and Witchcraft. In *Apachean Culture History and Ethnology.* Anthropological Papers of the University of Arizona. Number 21. Basso, Keith H. and Morris E. Opler, eds., pp. 91–114. Tucson: University of Arizona Press.

Larner, Christina
 1981   *Enemies of God. The Witch-hunt in Scotland.* London: Chatto and Windus.
Le Beau, Debie
 2002   Is Witchcraft Real? The Role of Perceptions in Health Seeking Behavior.
             In *Challenges for Anthropology in the "African Renaissance": A Southern
             African Contribution.* D. LeBeau and R.J. Gordon, eds., pp. 92–103.
             Windhoek: University of Namibia Press.
Leap, William L.
 1991   AIDS, Linguistics, and the Study of Non-Neutral Discourse in
             Anthropology, Sexuality and AIDS. *Journal of Sex Research* 28(2):275–88.
Leclerc-Madlala, Suzanne
 1997   Infect One, Infect All: Zulu Youth Response to the AIDS Epidemic in
             South Africa. *Medical Anthropology* 17:363–80.
 2001   Virginity Testing: Managing Sexuality in a Maturing HIV/AIDS
             Epidemic. *Medical Anthropology Quarterly* 15(4):533–52.
LeCompte, Margaret D., and Jean J. Schensul
 1999   *Analyzing and Interpreting Ethnographic Data.* Ethnographer's Toolkit 5.
             Walnut Creek, CA: AltaMira Press.
LeCompte, Margaret D., Jean J. Schensul, Margaret R. Weeks, and Merrill Singer
 1999   *Researcher Roles & Research Partnerships.* Ethnographer's Toolkit: 6.
             Walnut Creek, CA: AltaMira Press.
Lemert, Edwin M.
 1997   *The Trouble with Evil: Social Control at the Edge of Morality.* New York:
             State University of New York Press.
LeVine, Robert A.
 1982   *Culture, Behavior, and Personality: An Introduction to the Comparative Study
             of Psychosocial Adaptation.* New York: Aldine.
Levine, Susan and Fiona Ross
 2002   *Perceptions of and Attitudes to HIV/AIDS Among Young Adults at the
             University of Cape Town.* Center for Social Science Research Working
             Paper No. 14. Rondebosch: University of Cape Town.
Lewis, I. M.
 1970   A Structural Approach to Witchcraft and Spirit Possession. In *Witchcraft
             Confessions and Accusations.* Douglas, Mary, ed., pp. 293–309. London:
             Tavistock.
Lewis, O.
 1961   *The Children of Sanchez: Autobiography of a Mexican Family.* New York:
             Vintage Books.
Leiban, Richard W.
 1967   *Cebuano Sorcery: Malign Magic in the Philippines.* Berkeley: University of
             California Press.
Lindan, C., C. Allen, and M. Carael
 1991   Knowledge, Attitudes and Perceived Risk of AIDS Among Rwandan
             Women: Relationship to HIV Infection and Behavior Change. *AIDS*
             5:993–1002.

Linde, Paul R.
2002   *Of Spirits and Madness: An American Psychiatrist in Africa.* New York: McGraw-Hill.

Lindenbaum, Shirley
1981   Images of the Sorcerer in Papua New Guinea. *Social Analysis* 8:119–28.
1998   Images of Catastrophe: The Making of an Epidemic. In *The Political Economy of AIDS.* Merrill Singer, ed., pp. 33–58. Amityville, NY: Baywood Publishers.
2001   Kuru, Prions, and Human Affairs: Thinking About Epidemics. *Annual Review of Anthropology* 30:363–85.

Loeb, E. M.
1929   Shaman and Seer. *American Anthropologist* 31(1):60–84.

Loewenson, Rene, and Alan Whiteside
1997   *Social and Economic Issues of HIV/AIDS in Southern Africa.* SAfAIDS Occasional Paper Series: Volume 2. Harare: SAfAIDS.

Loudon, J. B.
1976   Preface. In *Social Anthropology and Medicine.* J.B. Loudon, ed., pp. v–viii. Association of Social Anthropologists Monograph, Vol. 13. London: Academic Press.

Loveless, J. H.
1918   Letter from the Wedza Reserve. In *Folder A3 12/30/1 Vol. 1.* Harare: National Archives of Zimbabwe.

Lush, Louisiana
2001   International Effort for Antiretrovirals: A Storm in a Teacup? *Tropical Medicine and International Health* 6(7):491–95.

Lussi, Kurt
2002   *Im Reich der Geister und tanzenden Hexen: Jenseitsvorstellungen, Dämonen und Zauberglaube.* Aarau: AT Verlag.

Mabuya, Precity
1998   Sethukile. In *Selections: Inkondlo.* Zimbabwe Women Writers, eds. P. 24. Harare: Zimbabwe Women Writers.

MacFarlane, Alan
1970   *Witchcraft in Tudor and Stuart England.* New York: Harper & Row.

Machein, Henning
1999   *AIDS, Wissen und Macht in Afrika: Zur Produktion von Wissen in der Aidsprävention in Mali.* M. A. Thesis. Department of African Studies. Köln: Institut für Afrikanistik Universität zu Köln.

MacLean, Sandra J.
2002   Mugabe at War: The Political Economy of Conflict in Zimbabwe. *Third World Quarterly* 23(3):513–28.

MacLean, William
1992   Racism, Poverty Fuel AIDS in South Africa. *The Chronicle* (Bulawayo). July 7. P. 2.

Madsen, William, and Claudia Madsen
1989   Mexico: Tecospa and Tepepan. In *Witchcraft and Sorcery of the American Native Peoples.* Walker, Deward E., ed., pp. 223–43. Moscow: Idaho.

Mafico, C. J. C.
    1989   *An Evaluation of Urban Planning Standards for Low Income Housing in Zimbabwe.* RUP Occasional Paper: Volume 21. Harare: Department of Rural and Urban Planning at the University of Zimbabwe.

Maines, David R.
    1999   Information Pools and Racialized Narrative Structures. *The Sociological Quarterly* 40(2):317–26.

Maingard, L. F.
    1929   *Some Linguistic Problems of South Africa. South African Journal of Science* 26(December):835–65.

Mair, Stefan, and Masipula Sithole
    2002   *Blocked Democracies in Africa: Case Study Zimbabwe.* Harare: Konrad Adenauer Foundation.

Makhobo, Dawn
    1989   AIDS in Africa. *Nursing RSA Vergleging* 4(3):20–22.

Makumbe, John, and Daniel Compagnon
    2000   *Behind the Smokescreen: The Politics of Zimbabwe's 1995 General Elections.* Harare: University of Zimbabwe Publications.

Makunike, Chido
    2003   Tendai Westerhof: Living Positively with AIDS. *The Financial Gazette* (Harare). March 6–12. P. 29.

Makuve, E. E.
    1991   Shameless Harlots of Borrowdale. *The Chronicle* (Bulawayo). October 5. P. 5.

Malinowski, Bronislaw
    1926   *Crime and Custom in Savage Society.* London: Routledge and Kegan-Paul.
    1943   The Pan-African Problem of Culture Contact (In Education and the Cultural Process). *American Journal of Sociology* 48: 649–65.
    1963   *Sex, Culture, and Myth.* London: Hart Davies.
    1969   Religion as a Social Function. In *Phenomenology of Religion: Eight Modern Descriptions of the Essence of Religion.* J. D. Bettis, ed., pp. 179–98. New York: Harper & Row.

Manderson, Leonore
    1998   Applying Medical Anthropology in the Control of Infectious Disease. *Tropical Medicine* 3(12):1020–27.

Manderson, Leonore, and P. Aaby
    1992   An Epidemic in the Field? Rapid Assessment Procedures and Health Research. *Social Science and Medicine* 35:839–50.

Mann, Jonathan M.
    1988   AIDS: A Global Strategy for a Global Challenge. *Impact of Science on Society* 150(39):159–67.

Marcus, Carin
    2002   *The Cultural Context of HIV/AIDS in South Africa.* M.A. Thesis, Social Work. Johannesburg: Rand Afrikaans University.

Marcus, George (ed.)
    1999   *Paranoia Within Reason: A Casebook on Conspiracy as Explanation.* Chicago: Chicago University Press.

Margolis, Eric
    1990   Visual Ethnography: Tools for Mapping the AIDS Epidemic. *Journal of*
                Contemporary Ethnography 19(3):370–91.

Marwick, Max
    1952   Another Modern Anti-Witchcraft Movement in East Central Africa.
                Africa 20(2):100–112.
    1963   The Sociology of Sorcery in a Central African Tribe. *African Studies*
                22(1):1–21.
    1965   *Sorcery in Its Social Setting: A Study of the Northern Rhodesian Cewa.*
                Manchester: Manchester University Press.
    1967   The Sociology of Sorcery in a Central African Tribe. In *Magic, Witchcraft,*
                and Curing. Middleton, J., ed., pp. 101–126. New York: The Natural
                History Press.
    1970   Sorcery as a "Social Strain-Gauge." In *Witchcraft and Sorcery: Selected*
                Readings. M. Marwick, ed., pp. 280–95. Harmondsworth: Penguin.

Mary Aquina, Sister O. P.
    1968   A Sociological Interpretation of Sorcery and Witchcraft Beliefs Among
                the Karanga. *NADA—The Rhodesia Ministry Internal Affairs Annual*
                9(5):47–51.

Mason, Fran
    2002   A Poor Person's Cognitive Mapping. In *Conspiracy Nation: The Politics of*
                Paranoia in Postwar America. P. Knight, ed., pp. 40–56. New York: New
                York University Press.

Masquelier, Adeline
    2000   Of Headhunters and Cannibals: Migrancy, Labor, and Consumption in
                the Mawri Imagination. *Cultural Anthropology* 15(1):84–126.
    2004   The Return of Magic. *Social Anthropology* 12(1):95–102.

Mathe, Lizwe
    1991   Abnormal Behavior. Letter to the Editor. *The Chronicle* (Bulawayo).
                October 11. P. 5.

Mavhungu, Khaukanani N.
    2002   Anthropology and African Witchcraft: Social "Strain-Gauge," Modernity
                and Witchcraft Violence in South Africa's Far-North. In *Challenges for*
                Anthropology in the "African Renaissance": A Southern African Contribution.
                D. LeBeau and R.J. Gordon, eds., pp. 68–79. Windhoek: University of
                Namibia Press.

Mayer, Phillip
    1970   Witches. In *Witchcraft and Sorcery: Selected Readings.* M. Marwick, ed.,
                pp. 45–64. Harmondsworth: Penguin Books.

Mays, V. M., and S. D. Cochran
    1996   Is there a Legacy of Tuskegee? AIDS Misbeliefs Among Inner-City
                African Americans and Hispanics. *International Conference on AIDS*
                11:190 (Abstract No. We. D. 3789).

McGary, H.
    1999   Distrust, Social Justice, and Health Care. *The Mount Sinai Journal of*
                Medicine 66:236–40.

McGrath, Janet W.
1992   The Biological Impact of Social Responses to the AIDS Epidemic. *Medical Anthropology* 15:63–79.

McGregor, JoAnn
1999   Containing Violence: Poisoning and Guerilla/Civilian Relations in Memories of Zimbabwe's Liberation War. In *Trauma and Life Stories: International Perspectives.* Kim Lacy Rogers, Selma Leydesdorff, and Graham Dawson, eds., pp. 13–159. London: Routledge.

McKinley, Robert
1982   Culture Meets Nature on the Six o'Clock News: An Example of American Cosmology. In *Researching American Culture: A Guide For Student Anthropologists.* C. P. Kottak, ed., pp. 75–86. Ann Harbor: University of Michigan Press.

McMillen, Heather
2004   The Adapting Healer: Pioneering Through Shifting Epidemiological and Sociocultural Landscapes. *Social Science and Medicine* 59:889–902.

Medina, Catherine Ketty
2002   *Predictors of HIV Testing in Low-Income, High-Risk Women of Color.* Ph.D. School of Arts and Sciences. Columbia University.

Medvedev, Zhores A.
1986   AIDS Virus Infection: A Soviet View of Its Origin. Letter to the Editor. *Journal of the Royal Society of Medicine* 79(8):494–95.

Meldrum, Andrew
2005   *Where We Have Hope: A Memoir of Zimbabwe.* New York: Atlantic Monthly Press.

Melley, Timothy
2000   *Empire of Conspiracy: The Culture of Paranoia in Postwar America.* Ithaca: Cornell University Press.
2002   Agency Panic and the Culture of Conspiracy. In *The Politics of Paranoia in Postwar America.* P. Knight, ed., pp. 57–81. New York: New York University Press.

Menegoni, Lorenza
1996   Conceptions of Tuberculosis and Therapeutic Choices in Highland Chiapas, Mexico. *Medical Anthropology Quarterly* 10(3):381–401.

Merkur, Daniel
1989   Arctic: Inuit. In *Witchcraft and Sorcery of the American Native Peoples.* Walker, Deward E., ed., pp. 11–21. Moscow: Idaho.

Meursing, Karla
1997   *A World of Silence: Living with AIDS in Matabeleland, Zimbabwe.* Amsterdam: Royal Tropical Institute.

Meursing, Karla, and Flora Sibindi
1999   HIV Counseling, A Luxury or Essential Need: Emotional, Social, and Informational Needs of Patients Diagnosed HIV-Positive in Zimbabwe. Manuscript, pp. 15.

Meyer, Birgit
    1995   *Translating the Devil: An African Appropriation of Pietist Protestantism: The Case of the Peki Ewe in Southeastern Ghana, 1847–1992.* Ph. D. Dissertation. University of Leiden.

Michelet, Jules
    1995   *Witchcraft, Sorcery, and Superstition.* New York: Carol Publishing Group.

Middleton, John
    1967   The Concept of "Bewitching" in Lugbara. In *Magic, Witchcraft, and Curing.* Middleton, John, ed., pp. 55–67. Garden City: Natural History Press.

Middleton, John, and E. H. Winter
    1963   Introduction. In *Witchcraft and Sorcery in East Africa.* J. Middleton and E.H. Winter, eds., pp. 1–26. New York: Frederick A. Praeger.

Ministry of Health and Child Welfare
    1999   Working Document for National AIDS Council Strategic Framework for a National Response to HIV/AIDS (2000–2004). Harare: Government Printer.

Ministry of Health and Child Welfare, and United Nations Program on HIV/AIDS.
    2003   *Zimbabwe National HIV/AIDS Estimates, 2003.* Harare: Government Printers.

Mitchell, J. Clyde
    1960   *The Meaning in Misfortune for Urban Africans. In African Systems of Thought.* M. Fortes and G. Dieterlen, eds., pp. 192–203. London: Oxford University Press.

Mlambo, Sharon
    1994   Love Potions Find a Ready Market. *The Chronicle* (Bulawayo). November 19. P. 4.

Mogensen, Overgaard Hanne
    1997   The Narrative of AIDS among the Tonga of Zambia. *Social Science & Medicine* 44(4):431–39.

Moore, Henrietta L., and Todd Sanders
    2001   Magical Interpretations and Material Realities: An Introduction. In *Magical Interpretations, Material Realities: Modernity, Witchcraft and the Occult in Postcolonial Africa.* H. L. Moore and S. Todd, eds., pp. 1–27. London: Routledge.

Moscovici, Serge
    1976   *La Psychoanalyse, Son Image et Son Public.* Paris: Presses Universitaires de France.
    1981   On Social Representations. In *Social Cognition: Perspectives on Everyday Understanding.* J.P. Forgas, ed. London: Academic Press.
    1984   The Phenomenon of Social Representations. In *Social Representations.* R. M. Farr, ed. Cambridge: Cambridge University Press.
    1987   The Conspiracy Mentality. In *Changing Conceptions of Conspiracy.* C. F. Graumann and S. Moscovici, eds., pp. 151–69. Springer Series in Social Psychology. New York: Springer-Verlag.

2001a   The History and Actuality of Social Representations. In *Social Representations: Explorations in Social Psychology*. S. Moscovici, ed., pp. 120–55. New York: New York University Press.

2001b   *Social Representations: Explorations in Social Psychology*. New York: New York University Press.

Moscovici, Serge, and Miles Hewstone

1983   Social Representations and Social Explanations: From the 'Naïve' to the 'Amateur' Scientist. In *Attribution Theory: Social and Functional Extensions*. M. Hewstone, ed., pp. 98–125. Oxford: Basil Blackwell.

Moscovici, Serge, and Georges Vignaux

2001   The Concept of Themata. In *Social Representations: Explorations in Social Psychology*. S. Moscovici, ed., pp. 156–83. New York: New York University Press.

Moyo, Sam, and John Makumbe

2000a   NGOs and development. In *NGOs, the State and Politics in Zimbabwe*. S. Moyo, J. Makumbe, and B. Raftopoulos, eds., pp. 7–70. Harare: Sapes Books.

2000b   The Socio-Economic Environment and NGOs. In *NGOs, the State and Politics in Zimbabwe*. S. Moyo, J. Makumbe, and B. Raftopoulos, eds., pp. 7–20. Harare: Sapes Books.

Mputu, Mbu

n. d.   Public Opinions on the Deadly Disease, Called AIDS, among the Members of the Sakata Tribe. Bandundu.

Msipa, Arnold

2004   Once the Best in Africa, Zimbabwe's Health System is Now in Shambles. Electronic Source: http://ipsnews.net. Last Accessed: February 13, 2005.

Mubvami, Takawira

1996   *Urban Poverty, Housing, and Municipal Governance in Zimbabwe*. Volume 3. Harare: Municipal Development Programme.

Mujokoro, Sandra

2003   Bulawayo Faces Severe Food Crisis. *The Daily News* (Harare). July 7. P. 5.

Mukumbira, Rodrick

2002   Women Accused of Bewitching AIDS Patients. *The Herald* (Harare). April 25. P. B 11.

Munk, Kirstine

1997   Traditional Healers, Traditional Hospitals and HIV/AIDS: A Case Study in KwaZulu-Natal. *AIDS Analysis Africa* 7(6):10–12.

Munodawafa, Davison, and Clement Gwede

1996   Patterns of HIV/AIDS in Zimbabwe: Implications for Health Education. *AIDS Education and Prevention* 8(1):1–10.

Munthali, Joshua

1996   Undertakers Make a Killing from Dying. *The Chronicle* (Bulawayo). January 3. P. 4.

Munyavi, Sam

1990   Dicing with Death. *The Herald* (Harare). October 17. P. 2.

Mupedziswa, Rodreck
    1998   *AIDS in Africa: The Social Work Response.* Harare: School of Social Work.
Murray, Gerald F., and Maria Dolores Alvarez
    1973   Childbearing, Sickness and Healing in a Haitian Village, pp. 103. New York: Division of Social and Administrative Sciences; International Institute for the Study of Human Reproduction; Columbia University.
Mutandwa, Andrew
    1996   AIDS Can't Be Spread by the Mubobobo. *The Herald* (Harare). June 20. P. 12.
Mutasa, Salatiel
    2003a   AIDS Patients, A Forgotten Lot. *The Chronicle* (Bulawayo). October 30. P. 4.
    2003b   Funeral Expenses Beyond Reach of Many. *The Chronicle* (Bulawayo). October 18. P. 2.
    2003c   Hard Times for Health Sector. *The Chronicle* (Bulawayo). October 22. P. 4.
Mutemi, Arnold
    2003   Orphans Fail to Write Exam: $ 8 Billion Funds Lie Idle, DAACs Given 60 Days to Account for All Monies. *The Chronicle* (Bulawayo). August 15. P. 1.
Mutizwa-Mangiza, Dorothy
    1999   *Doctors and the State: The Struggle for Professional Control in Zimbabwe.* Brookfield VT: Aldershot.
Mwanza, Allast
    1999   *Social Policy in an Economy under Stress: The Case of Zimbabwe.* Harare: Sapes Books.
Nadel, S. F.
    1970   Witchcraft in Four African Societies. In *Witchcraft and Sorcery: Selected Readings.* M. Marwick, ed., pp. 264–79. Harmondsworth: Penguin Books.
Nangati, Fanuel
    1991   ZINATHA Community Based Health Education Programme on HIV/AIDS: Report on Knowledge, Attitudes, and Practices of Traditional Healers (Gutu District Baseline Survey), pp. 46. Harare.
National AIDS Council
    2003   AIDS: A National Crisis Calling for Accountability and Transparency. *The Chronicle* (Bulawayo). May 20, pp. 32.
Nations, Marilyn, and Cristina Monte
    1997   I'm No Dog, No!: Cries of Resistance against Cholera Control Campaigns in Brazil. In *The Anthropology of Infectious Disease: International Health Perspectives.* M. C. Inhorn and P. J. Brown, eds., pp. 439–81. Amsterdam: Gordon and Breach.
Ncube, Cornelious Mayuyu
    2003   Mystery Surrounds Origins of Cancer. *The Chronicle* (Bulawayo). August 16. P. 6.
Ndhlukula, N. P.
    1980   *Imvelo Lolimi LweSiNdebele.* Gweru (Zimbabwe): Mambo Press.

Ndlovu, Gwakuba Saul
2003a   Homosexuality Is No Doubt Ungodly. *The Daily News* (Harare).
           September 11, p. 10.
Ndlovu, Rose, and Ruth Sihlangu
1992   Preferred Sources of Information on AIDS among High School Students
           from Selected Schools in Zimbabwe. Journal of Advanced Nursing
           17:507–513.
Ndlovu, Sinqobile
2003b   Do Men Who Always Feel Sleepy Suffer from Sleeping Sickness? *The
           Chronicle* (Bulawayo). August 16. P. 9.
Ndubani, Phillimon
1998   *Death, Witchcraft, and AIDS: A Review of the Current Situation and
           Perceptions among the Goba People of Chiawa Chieftaincy, Rural Zambia.*
           Lusaka: University of Zambia.
Ndubiwa, Mike
1972   *African Participation in Housing Management in Rhodesia: The Bulawayo
           African Advisory Board.* Master of Social Science. Local Government and
           Administration. University of Birmingham.
1974   *Bulawayo Municipal African Townships.* Occasional Paper: Volume 2.
           Bulawayo: City Housing and Amenities Department.
Nelkin, Dorothy, and Sander Gilman
1991   Placing Blame for Devastating Disease. In *In Time of Plague: The History
           and Social Consequences of Lethal Epidemic Disease.* A. Mack, ed. New
           York: New York University Press.
Ngubane, Harriet
1976   Some Aspects of Treatment among the Zulu. In *Social Anthropology
           and Medicine.* J.B. Loudon, ed., pp. 318–57. Association of Social
           Anthropologists of the Commonwealth Monograph, Vol. 13. London:
           Academic Press.
Nicholas, Lionel, and Kevin Durrheim
1995   Religiosity, AIDS, and Sexuality: Attitudes, Belief, and Practices of
           Black South African First Year University Students. *Psychological Reports*
           77:1328–30.
Nicoll, A., U. Laukamm-Josten, B. Mwizarubi, C. Mayala, M. Mkuye, G. Nyembela, and
H. Grosskurth
1993   Lay Health Beliefs Concerning HIV and AIDS, A Barrier for Control
           Programmes. *AIDS Care* 5(2):231–40.
Niehaus, Isak
2001   *Witchcraft, Power, and Politics: Exploring the Occult in the South African
           Lowveld, Anthropology, Culture, and Society.* London: Pluto Press.
Niehaus, Isak and Gunvor Jonsson
2005   Dr. Wouter Basson, Americans, and Wild Beasts: Men's Conspiracy
           Theories on HIV/AIDS in the South African Lowveld. *Medical
           Anthropology* 24:179–208.

Niles, John D.
  1999   *Homo Narrans: The Poetics and Anthropology of Oral Literature.*
              Philadelphia: University of Pennsylvania Press.
Nkala, Nomsa
  1999   HIV Patients Die after Alleged Experiments. *The Herald* (Harare).
              October 16. P. 1.
Nkala, Oscar
  2003   Gukurahundi Ghosts Rise Again. *The Daily News* on Sundays (Harare).
              July 13. P. 4.
Nkomo, Ntungamili
  2003a   90 Percent of Zimbabweans Languish in Poverty. *The Daily News*
              (Harare). July 17. P. 18.
  2003b   Fuel Shortages Hit Food Aid Distribution. *The Daily News* (Harare).
              August 2. P. 3.
Noireau, F.
  1987   HIV Transmission from Monkey to Man. Letter to the Editor. *The Lancet*
              (June 27):1498–99.
Nowak, Michael, and Juha Kähkönen
  2004   Zimbabwe: 2004 Article IV Consultation, Staff Report, pp. 58.
              Washington, DC: International Monetary Fund.
Nyathi, Thembeni
  1998   I-AIDS. In *Selections: Inkondlo.* Zimbabwe Women Writers, eds. p. 31.
              Harare: Zimbabwe Women Writers.
Nyikadzino, L. A.
  1991   The Truth about AIDS. Letter to the Editor. *The Chronicle* (Bulawayo).
              March 4. P. 5.
Nzenza-Shand, Sekai
  1997   *Songs to an African Sunset: A Zimbabwean Story.* Melbourne: Lonely Planet
              Publications.
Obeyesekere, Gananath
  1975   Sorcery, Premeditated Murder, and the Canalization of Aggression in Sri
              Lanka. *Ethnology* 14(1):1–23.
Offiong, Daniel A.
  1991   *Witchcraft, Sorcery, Magic and Social Order among the Ibibio of Nigeria.*
              Enugu, Nigeria: Fourth Dimension Publishing.
Palmiere, Andrew
  2000   *The Social and Economic Impacts of HIV/AIDS on High-Density Households
              in Bulawayo, Zimbabwe.* M.A. Geography. University of Calgary.
Palmiere, Andrew, and Miriam Grant
  2001   Unequal Balance: HIV/AIDS and Health Care Programmes in Bulawayo,
              Zimbabwe. *South African Historical Journal* 45(November):154–77.
Parish, Jane
  2001   The Age of Anxiety. In *The Age of Anxiety: Conspiracy Theory and the Human
              Sciences.* J. Parish and M. Parker, eds., pp. 1–16. Oxford: Blackwell.
Park, Willard Z.
  1934   Paviotso Shamanism. *American Anthropologist* 36(1):98–113.

Parker, Martin
    2001   Human Science as Conspiracy Theory. In *The Age of Anxiety: Conspiracy Theory and the Human Sciences*. J. Parish and M. Parker, eds., pp. 191–207. Oxford: Blackwell Publishers.

Parrinder, Geoffrey
    1963   *Witchcraft: European and African*. London: Faber and Faber.

Parsons, S., W. Simmons, F. Shinhoster, and J. Kilburn
    1999   A Test of the Grapevine: An Empirical Examination of Conspiracy Theories among African Americans. *Sociological Spectrum* 19(2):201–222.

Pasteur, David
    1994   From Frontier Town Board to Modern Municipality: A Hundred Years of Local Government in Bulawayo. In *100 Years of Industry in Bulawayo: 1894–1994*, pp. 78–119. Bulawayo: Matabeleland Chamber of Industries.

Patel, Diana
    1988   Some Issues of Urbanization and Development in Zimbabwe. *Journal of Social Development in Africa* 3(2):17–31.

Patterson, M.
    1974/75   Sorcery and Witchcraft in Melanesia. *Oceania* 45:132–60;212–34.

Patton, Michael Quinn
    1990   *Qualitative Evaluation and Research Methods*. Newbury Park: Sage Publications.

Pelling, Margaret
    1993   Contagion/Germ Theory/Specificity. In *Companion Encyclopedia of the History of Medicine*. Volume 1. W. F. Bynum and R. Porter, eds., pp. 309–334. London: Routledge.

Pels, Peter
    2003   Introduction: Magic and Modernity. In *Magic and Modernity: Interfaces of Revelation and Concealment*. B. Meyer and P. Pels, eds., pp. 1–38. Stanford: Stanford University Pres.

Pelto, Pertti J., and Gretel H. Pelto
    1978   *Anthropological Research: The Structure of Inquiry*. Cambridge: Cambridge University Press.

Pelton, Mary Helen and Jacqueline DiGennaro
    1992   *Images of a People: Tlingit Myths and Legends*. Englewood: Libraries Unlimited.

Percival, Lynda J., and Vimla Patel
    n. d.   Sexual Beliefs and Practices by Women in Urban Zimbabwe, pp. 17. Montreal.

Perice, Glen A.
    1997   Rumors and Politics in Haiti. *Anthropological Quarterly* 70(1):1–10.

Pfeiffer, James
    2004   Condom Social Marketing, Pentecostalism, and Structural Adjustment in Mozambique: A Clash of AIDS Prevention Messages. *Medical Anthropology Quarterly* 18(1):77–103.

Phillips, Howard
    1990   "*Black October*": *The Impact of the Spanish Influenza Epidemic of 1918 on South Africa*. Pretoria: The Government Printer.

Phiri, Virginia
    1998   Isililo Esibi. In *Selections: Inkondlo*. Zimbabwe Women Writers, eds., p. 32. Harare: Zimbabwe Women Writers.

Pipes, Daniel
    1996   *The Hidden Hand: Middle East Fears of Conspiracy*. New York: St. Martin's Press.
    1997   *Conspiracy: How the Paranoid Style Flourishes and Where It Comes From*. New York: The Free Press.

Pitts, Marian
    1990   Attitudes, Knowledge, Experiences and Behavior Related to HIV and AIDS among Zimbabwean Social Workers. *AIDS Care* 2(1):53–61.

Pitts, Marian, Moira Humphrey, and Paul Wilson
    1991   Assessments of Personal and General Risks of HIV and AIDS in Harare, Zimbabwe. *Health and Education Research* 6(3):307–311.

Pitts, Marian, and Helen Jackson
    1993a   No Joking Matter: Formal and Informal Sources of Information About AIDS in Zimbabwe. AIDS Education and Prevention 5(3):212–19.
    1993b   Press Coverage of AIDS in Zimbabwe: A Five Year Review. *AIDS Care* 5(2):223–30.

Pócs, Eva
    1999   *Between the Living and the Dead: A Perspective on Witches and Seers in the Early Modern Age*. Budapest: Central European University Press.

Pollock, Donald
    1996   Personhood and Illness among the Kulina. *Medical Anthropology Quarterly* 10(3):319–41.

Popper, Karl R.
    1962   *Conjectures and Refutations: The Growth of Scientific Knowledge*. New York: Basic Books.
    1966   *The Open Society and Its Enemies (Volume 2): The High Tide of Prophecy: Hegel, Marx, and the Aftermath*. London: Routledge and Kegan Paul.

Porter, Michael
    2001   *The Conspiracy to Destroy Black Women*. Chicago: African American Images.

Porter, Roy
    1993   Religion and Medicine. In *Companion Encyclopedia of the History of Medicine. Volume 2*. W. F. Bynum and R. Porter, eds., pp. 1449–68. London: Routledge.

Price-Smith, Andrew T., and John L. Daly
    2004   *Downward Spiral: HIV/AIDS, State Capacity, and Political Conflict in Zimbabwe*. Peaceworks: Volume 53. Washington, DC: United States Institute of Peace.

Prinz, Armin
    1998   "Kaza Basolo"—A Culture-Bound Syndrome Among the Azande of Northeast-Congo. *Curare* 14(Sonderheft):53–57.

2001   "Kaza Basolo"—A Culture-Bound Syndrome Among the Azande of
Northeast-Congo. *Viennese Ethnomedicine Newsletter* 4(1):12, 16–19.

Raftopoulos, Brian
2001   The Labor Movement and the Emergence of Opposition Politics in
Zimbabwe. In *Striking Back: The Labor Movement and the Post-Colonial
State in Zimbabwe 1980–2000.* B. Raftopoulos and L. Sachikonye, eds.,
pp. 1–24. Harare: Weaver Press.

Raftopoulos, Brian, Tony Hawkins, and Dede Amanor-Wilks
1998   *The Zimbabwe Human Development Report.* Harare: UNDP, UNICEF, IDS,
Poverty Reduction Forum.

Rakwar, J., N. Kidula, K. Fonck, P. Kirui, J. Ndinya-Achola, and M. Temmerman
1999   HIV/STD: The Women to Blame? Knowledge and Attitudes Among
STD Clinic Attendees in the Second Decade of HIV/AIDS. *International
Journal of STD and AIDS* 10:543–47.

Ramadu
2001   Ingculaza. In *Izambulelo: Traditional Contemporary Music from Zimbabwe.*
Compact Disc. Graz: Neue Welt Studios.

Randall-David, Betsy
1987   Adolescents' Attitudes, Knowledge and Beliefs about AIDS. Conference
on Theoretical Issues in AIDS Social Research, Minneapolis, Minnesota,
1987.

Ranger, Terence O.
1991   Religion and Witchcraft in Everyday Life in Contemporary Zimbabwe.
In *Cultural Struggle and Development in Southern Africa.* P. Kaarsholm, ed.,
pp. 149–65. London: James Currey.
1999   *Voices from the Rocks: Nature, Culture and History in the Matopos Hills of
Zimbabwe.* Harare: Baobab.

Ransford, Oliver
1968   *Bulawayo: Historic Battleground of Rhodesia.* Cape Town: A. A. Balkema.

Rasmussen, R. Kent, and Steven C. Rubert
1990   *Historical Dictionary of Zimbabwe. African Historical Dictionaries: Volume
46.* Metuchen: The Scarecrow Press.

Reay, Marie
1987a   The Magico-Religious Foundations of New Guinea Highlands Warfare.
In *Sorcerer and Witch in Melanesia.* Stephen, Michelle, ed., pp. 83–120.
New Brunswick: Rutgers University Press.
1987b   *The Kuma: Freedom and Conformity in the New Guinea Highlands.* New
Haven: Yale University Press.

Redmayne, Alison
1970   Chikanga: An African Diviner with an International Reputation. In
Witchcraft Confessions and Accusations. Douglas, Mary, ed., pp. 103–128.
London: Tavistock.

Revilo
2003   Zimbabwe Beautiful Flower Left to Wilt. *The Daily News* (Harare).
August 11. P. 9.

Reynolds, Pamela
    1990   Zezuru Turn of the Screw: On Children's Exposure to Evil. *Culture, Medicine, and Psychiatry* 14(3):313–37.

Richardson, L.
    1997   Experiment Leaves Legacy of Distrust of New AIDS Drugs. *The New York Times.* April 21. P. A1.

Robbins, Michael, and Justin M. Nolan
    2000   A Measure of Semantic Category Clustering in Free-Listing Tasks. *Field Methods* 12(1):18–28.

Robins, Robert S., and Jerrold M. Post
    1997   *Political Paranoia: The Psychopolitics of Hatred.* New Haven: Yale University Press.

Robinson, Noah Jamie, and Rav Marindo
    1999   Current Estimates of and Future Projections for Adult Deaths Attributed to HIV Infection in Zimbabwe. *Journal of Acquired Immune Deficiency Syndromes and Human Retrovirology* 20:187–94.

Rödlach, Alexander
    2004   Women, Dogs, and Sex: How to Make Sense of Statements on HIV/AIDS in Bulawayo, Zimbabwe. *AIDS and Anthropology Bulletin* 16(1):4–7.
    2005   *Blaming "Others" for HIV/AIDS in an Urban Township in Bulawayo, Zimbabwe: Witchcraft Beliefs and Conspiracy Suspicions.* Ph.D. Dissertation, Department of Anthropology. Gainesville: University of Florida.
    in press   Apocalyse Now! Interpretations of HIV/AIDS in an Urban Township in Bulawayo, Zimbabwe. In *Cosmologies of Suffering.* Lazar, Imre and Agita Luse (eds.). Newcastle-upon-Tyne: Cambridge Scholars Press.

Rodman, Julius Scammon
    1979   *The Kahuna Sorcerers of Hawaii, Past and Present.* Hicksville NY: Exposition Press.

Romanucci-Ross, Lola
    1977   The Hierarchy of Resort in Curative Practices: The Admirality Islands, Melanesia. In *Culture, Disease, and Healing: Studies in Medical Anthropology.* David Landy, ed., pp. 481–87. New York: Macmillan.

Romberg, Raquel
    2003   *Witchcraft and Welfare: Spiritual Capital and the Business of Magic in Modern Puerto Rico.* Austin: University of Texas Press.

Romero-Daza, Nancy
    1994   Multiple Sexual Partners, Migrant Labor, and the Makings for an Epidemic: Knowledge and Beliefs About AIDS Among Women in Highland Lesotho. *Human Organization* 53(2):192–205.
    1995   Design of HIV Awareness Materials in Rural Costa Rica: A Community Participatory Approach. AIDS and Anthropology Bulletin 17(2):23–25.

Roos, Gun
    1998   Pile Sorting: "Kids Like Candy." In *Using Methods in the Field: A Practical Introduction and Casebook.* V. C. de Munck and E. J. Sobo, eds., pp. 97–110. Walnut Creek: AltaMira Press.

Rotberg, Robert I.
2002   *Ending Autocracy, Enabling Democracy: The Tribulations of Southern Africa,
          1960–2000.* Washington, DC: Brookings Institution Press.
Rutherford, Blair
1999   To Find an African Witch: Anthropology, Modernity, and Witch-Finding
          in North-West Zimbabwe. *Critique of Anthropology* 19(1):89–109.
Sabatier, Renée
1987   *AIDS and the Third World.* London: The Panos Institute.
Sabatier, Renée, and Jon Tinker
1988   *Blaming Others: Prejudice, Race, and Worldwide AIDS.* Washington: Panos
          Institute.
Sahagún, Fray Bernardino de
1981   *Historia General de las Cosas de Nueva España.* Angel Maria Garibay K.,
          ed. Mexico City: Editorial Porrúa.
Salamon, Frank
1983   Shamanism and Politics in Late-Colonial Ecuador. *American Ethnologist*
          10(3):413–28.
Saler, Benson
1964   Nagual, Witch, and Sorcerer in a Quiché Village. *Ethnology* 3:305–28.
Saller, Karla
2004   *The Judicial Institution in Zimbabwe.* Cape Town: Siber Ink.
Sanders, Todd, and Harry G. West
2003   Powers Revealed and Concealed in the New World Order. In
          *Transparency and Conspiracy: Ethnographies of Suspicion in the New World
          Order.* H. G. West and T. Sanders, eds., pp. 1–37. Durham: Duke
          University Press.
Sankara, Thomas
1995   Witches Blamed for AIDS in the Congo. *AIDS Analysis Africa* (August):3.
Sasson, Theodore
1995   African-American Conspiracy Theories and the Social Construction of
          Crime. *Sociological Inquiry* 65(3-4):265–85.
Scaletta, Naomi M.
1985   Death by Sorcery: The Social Dynamics of Dying in Bariai, West New
          Britain. In *Aging and its Transformations: Moving Toward Death in Pacific
          Societies.* Ayers-Counts, Dorothy and David R. Counts, eds., pp. 223–47.
          Pittsburgh: University of Pittsburgh Press.
Schapera, Isaac
1970   Sorcery and Witchcraft in Bechuanaland. In *Witchcraft and Sorcery:
          Selected Readings.* M. Marwick, ed., pp. 108–20. Harmondsworth:
          Penguin Books.
Schensul, Stephen L.., Jean J. Schensul, and Margaret D. LeCompte
1999   *Essential Ethnographic Methods: Observations, Interviews, and Questionnaires.*
          Ethnographer's Toolkit 2. Walnut Creek, CA: AltaMira Press.
Schmitt, Ellen
1999   *AIDS und Gesellschaft in Zimbabwe: Eine Qualitative Untersuchung.* Beiträge
          zur Ethnomedizin: Volume 3. Berlin: Verlag für Wissenschaft und Bildung.

Schneider, Helen and Didier Fassin
    2002   Denial and Defiance: A Socio-Political Analysis of AIDS in South Africa. *AIDS* 16(Supplement 4):S45–S51.

Schoepf, Brooke G.
    1991   Ethical, Methodological, and Political Issues of AIDS Research in Central Africa. *Social Science and Medicine* 33(7):749–63.
    1995   Culture, Sex Research, and AIDS Prevention in Africa. In *Culture and Sexual Risk: Anthropological Perspectives on AIDS.* H. ten Brummelhuis and G. Herdt, eds., pp. 29–51. Amsterdam: Gordon and Breach.
    2001   International AIDS Research in Anthropology: Taking a Critical Perspective on the Crisis. *Annual Review of Anthropology* 61:335–61.

Scholz-Williams, Gerhild
    1995   *Defining Dominion: The Discourses of Magic and Witchcraft in Early Modern France and Germany.* Ann Arbor: University of Michigan Press.

Schoormann, Matthias
    2005   *Sozialer und religiöser Wandel in Afrika: Die Tonga in Zimbabwe.* Serie Kulturelle Identität und politische Selbstbestimmung in der Weltgesellschaft, Band 11. Münster: Lit Verlag.

Schrauwers, Albert
    2003   Through a Glass Darkly: Charity, Conspiracy, and Power in New Order Indonesia. In *Transparency and Conspiracy: Ethnographies of Suspicion in the New World Order.* West, Harry G, and Todd Sanders, eds., pp. 125–47. Durham: Duke University Press.

Scogings, F.
    1918   Letter from the Mangeni Native Reserve. In *Folder A3 12/30/1 Vol. 1.* Harare: National Archives of Zimbabwe.

Scott, James
    1985   *Weapons of the Weak: Everyday Forms of Peasant Resistance.* New Haven: Yale University Press.

Scott, Sally, and Mary Mercer
    1994   Understanding Cultural Obstacles to HIV/AIDS Prevention in Africa. *AIDS Education and Prevention* 6(1):81–89.

Segal, Jakob
    1990   *AIDS: Die Spur führt ins Pentagon.* Essen: Verlag Neuer Weg.

Segar, Julia
    1997a   Hard Lives and Evil Winds: Illness Aetiology and the Search for Healing among Ciskeian Villagers. *Social Science & Medicine* 44(10):1585–1600.
    1997b   The Pursuit of Health in a Keishammahoek Village. In *From Reserve to Region: Apartheid and Social Change in the Keishammerhoek District of (former) Ciskei, 1950–1990.* C. de Wet and M. Whisson, eds., pp. 186–223. Grahamstown: Rhodes University.

Selby, Henry
    1974   *Zapotec Deviance: The Convergence of Folk and Modern Sociology.* Austin: University of Texas Press.

Sengupta, Sohini, and Ronald P Strauss, Robert deVellis, Sandra Crouse Quinn, Brenda deVellis, William B. Ware.
    2000   Factors Affecting African-American Participation in AIDS research. *Journal of Acquired Immune Deficiency Syndromes* 24(3):275–84.

Setel, Phillip
    1999   *A Plague of Paradoxes: AIDS, Culture, and Demography in Northern Tanzania.* Chicago: University of Chicago Press.

Shelley, Gene Ann
    1992   *The Social Networks of People with End Stage Renal Disease: Comparing Hemodialysis and Peritoneal Dialysis Patients.* Ph.D. Dissertation. Anthropology. University of Florida.

Shelley, Wilfred
    1918   Report from Fr. Wilfred Shelley of St. Augustine's Mission in Penhalonga to the Chief Native Commissioner in Salisbury from the 17th of December 1918. In *Folder A3 12/30/1 Vol. 1.* Harare: National Archives.

Schensul, Jean J.
    1998   Organizing Community Research Partnerships in the Struggle Against AIDS. *Health Education and Behavior* 26(2):266–83.

Sibanda, Amson
    2000   A Nation in Pain: Why the HIV Epidemic Is Out of Control in Zimbabwe. *International Journal of Health Services* 30(4):717–38.

Sidky, H.
    1997   *Witchcraft, Lycanthropy, Drugs, and Disease: An Anthropological Study of the European Witch-Hunts.* New York: Peter Lang.

Siegel, James T.
    2003   The Truth of Sorcery. *Cultural Anthropology* 18(2):135–55.

Siegel, Karolynn, and Laurie J. Bauman
    1986   Methodological Issues in AIDS-Related Research. In *The Social Dimensions of AIDS: Method and Theory.* D.A. Feldman and T. M. Johnson, eds., pp. 15–39. New York: Praeger.

Sigerist, Henry E.
    1951   *A History of Medicine: Primitive and Archaic. Volume 1.* Oxford: Oxford University Press.

Silverblatt, Irene
    1987   *Moon, Sun, and Witches.* Princeton: Princeton University Press.

Simmons, David Sean
    2002   *Managing Misfortune: HIV/AIDS, Health Development, and Traditional Healers in Zimbabwe.* Ph. D. Dissertation. Department of Anthropology. Michigan State University.

Sindzingre, N.
    1995   The Need for Meaning, the Explanation of Ill Fortune: The Senufo. In *The Meaning of Illness: The Anthropology, History, and Sociology of Illness.* M. Auge and C. Herzlich, eds., pp. 71–96. Luxembourg: Harwood Academic.

Singer, Merrill
    1995   Beyond the Ivory Tower: Critical Praxis in Medical Anthropology. *Medical Anthropology Quarterly* 9(1):80–106.

Skinner, Jonathan
    2001   Taking Conspiracy Seriously: Fantastic Narratives and Mr. Grey the Pan-Africanist on Montserrat. In *The Age of Anxiety: Conspiracy Theory and the Human Sciences.* J. Parish and M. Parker, eds., pp. 93–111. Oxford: Blackwell.

Skold, Reverend
    1918   Report of Reverend Skold of the Church of Sweden Mission in Belingwe to the Native Commissioner in Belingwe. In *Folder A3 12/30/1 Vol. 1.* Harare: National Archives.

Smith, C.
    1999   African Americans and the Medical Establishment. *The Mount Sinai Journal of Medicine* 66:280–81.

Smith, Laura C., Kenya J. Lucas, and Carl Latkin
    1999   Rumor and Gossip: Social Discourses on HIV and AIDS. *Anthropology & Medicine* 6(1):121–31.

Sobo, Elisa
    1995   *Choosing Unsafe Sex: AIDS Risk Denial Among Disadvantaged Women.* Philadelphia: University of Pennsylvania Press.

Sontag, Susan
    1990   *Illness as Metaphor and AIDS and Its Metaphors.* New York: Anchor Books.

Spindler, Louise
    1989   Great Lakes: Menomini. In *Witchcraft and Sorcery of the American Native Peoples.* Walker, Deward E., ed., pp. 39–74. Moscow: Univeristy of Idaho Press.

Spittler, Gerd
    2001   Teilnehmende Beobachtung als Dichte Teilnahme. *Zeitschrift für Ethnologie* 126:1–25.

Spradley, James P.
    1979   *The Ethnographic Interview.* New York: Holt.

Stadler, Jonathan
    2003   Rumor, Gossip and Blame: Implications for HIV/AIDS Prevention in the South African Lowveld. *Aids Education and Prevention* 15(4):357–68.

Stally, Aulora
    2000   SAfAIDS Media Training Workshop on HIV/AIDS. Harare: Southern African AIDS Information Dissemination Service.

Stamps, Timothy
    1999   Ministerial Statement on AIDS. In *Ministerial Statements of the Parliament of Zimbabwe from the 16th of March 1999, 4710–37.*

Stansbury, James P., and Manuel Sierra
    2004   Risks, Stigma and Honduran Garífuna Conceptions of HIV/AIDS. *Social Science & Medicine* 59:457–71.

Steadman, Lyle B.
    1985   The Killing of Witches. *Oceania* 56(2):106–123.

Stephen, Michelle
    1987a   Introduction. In *Sorcerer and Witch in Melanesia.* Stephen, Michelle, ed., pp. 1–14. New Brunswick: Rutgers University Press.

1987b   Master of Souls: The Mekeo Sorcerer. In *Sorcerer and Witch in Melanesia.* Stephen, Michelle, ed., pp. 41–80. New Brunswick: Rutgers University Press.

Stevens, Phillips
1996   Sorcery and Witchcraft. In *Encyclopedia of Cultural Anthropology.* D. Levinson and M. Ember, eds., pp. 1225–32, Vol. 4. New York: Henry Holt.

Stewart, Pamela, and Andrew Strathern
2004   *Witchcraft, Sorcery, Rumors, and Gossip.* Cambridge: Cambridge University Press.

Strecker, Robert
1986   AIDS Virus Infection. Letter to the Editor. *Journal of the Royal Society of Medicine,* pp. 560–61.

Strunin, L., and R. Hingson
1987   Acquired Immunodeficiency Syndrome and Adolescents: Knowledge, Beliefs, Attitudes and Behaviors. *Pediatrics* 79(5):825–28.

Sweet, James H.
2003   *Recreating Africa: Culture, Kinship, and Religion in the African-Portuguese World, 1441–1770.* Chapel Hill: University of North Carolina Press.

Taussig, Michael
1980   *The Devil and Commodity Fetishism in South America.* Chapel Hill: University of North Carolina Press.
1987   *Shamanism, Colonialism, and the Wild Man: A Study in Terror and Healing.* Chicago: University of Chicago Press.
1992   *The Nervous System.* London: Routledge.

Taylor, Christopher C.
1990   AIDS and the Pathogenesis of Metaphor. In *Culture and AIDS.* D. Feldman, ed., pp. 55–65. New York: Praeger.

Taylor, C.
1992   *Milk, Honey, and Money: Changing Concepts in Rwandan Healing.* Washington, D.C.: Smithsonian Institution Press.

Tembo, T., and Kupe
2002   Health Delivery System and the Drought Situation. In *The Humanitarian Situation in Zimbabwe: Private Sector & Civil Society Perspective—Mapping a Way Forward.* P. R. Forum and I. o. D. Studies, eds., pp. 11–13. Harare: Poverty Reduction Forum, Institute of Development Studies.

Thomas, Stephen B., and James W. Curran
1999   Tuskegee: From Science to Conspiracy to Metaphor. *The American Journal of the Medical Sciences* 317(1):1–4.

Thomas, Stephen B., and Sandra Crouse Quinn
1991   The Tuskegee Syphilis Study, 1932–1972: Implications for HIV Education and AIDS Risk Education Programs in the Black Community. *American Journal of Public Health* 81:1498–1505.

Thomas Aquinas, Saint
1947   *The Summa Theologica.* Translated by Fathers of the English Dominican Province. New York: Benziger Bros.

Thomas Aquinas, Saint *(continued)*
> 1975   *Summa Contra Gentiles. Book One: God.* Translated, with an Introduction and Notes, by Anton C. Pegis. Notre Dame: University of Notre Dame Press.

Tillotson, Jonathan, and Pranitha Maharaj
> 2001   Barriers to HIV/AIDS Protective Behavior Among African Adolescent Males in Township Secondary Schools in Durban, South Africa. *Society in Transition* 32(1):83–100.

Treichler, Paula A.
> 1989   AIDS and HIV Infection in the Third World: A First World Chronicle. In *Remaking History.* B. Kruger and P. Mariani, eds., pp. 31–86. Seattle: Bay Press.
> 1999   *How to Have a Theory in an Epidemic: Cultural Chronicles of AIDS.* Durham: Duke University Press.

Trotter, Robert T.
> 1991   Ethnographic Research Methods for Applied Medical Anthropology. In *Training Manual in Applied Medical Anthropology.* C. E. Hill, ed., pp. 180–212. Washington, D.C.: American Anthropological Association.

Tule, Philipus
> 2004   *Longing for the House of God, Dwelling in the House of the Ancestors.* Studia Instituti Anthropos, Volume 50. Fribourg: Academic Press.

Turner, Castellano, and William A. Darity
> 1973   Fears of Genocide Among Black Americans as Related to Age, Sex, and Region. *American Journal of Public Health* 63:1029–34.

Turner, Patricia A.
> 1993   *I Heard It Through the Grapevine: Rumor in African American Culture.* Berkeley: University of California Press.

Turner, Victor
> 1964   Witchcraft and Sorcery: Taxonomy Versus Dynamics. *Africa* 34(4):314–24.
> 1968   *The Drums of Affliction: A Study of Religious Processes among the Ndembu of Zambia.* Oxford: Clarendon Press.
> 1981   *The Drums of Affliction: A Study of Religious Processes among the Ndembu of Zambia.* Ithaca: Cornell University Press.

UNAIDS and World Health Organization
> 2004   Epidemiological Fact Sheet on HIV/AIDS and Sexually Transmitted Infections: Zimbabwe 2004 Update. Electronic Source: http://www.unaids.org. Last accessed: November 28, 2004.

van Binsbergen, Wim
> 1981   Religious Change and the Problem of Evil in Western Zambia. In *Religious Change in Zambia: Exploratory Studies.* W. van Binsbergen, ed., pp. 593–614. London: Kegan Paul International.

van den Borne, Francine
> *2005*   *Trying to Survive in Times of Poverty and AIDS: Women and Multiple Partner Sex in Malawi.* Series Health, Culture, and Society: Studies in Medical Anthropology and Sociology. Amsterdam: Het Spinhuis.

van der Drift, Roy
    1992   *Arbeid en Alcohol: De Dynamiek van de Rijstverbouw en het Gezag van de Outsten bij de Balanta Brassa in Guinee Bissau.* Leiden: Research School of Asian, African, and Amerindian Studies (CNWS).

van Onselen, C.
    1972   Reactions to Rinderpest in Southern Africa: 1896-1897. *Journal of African History* 13(3):473–88.

Vankin, Jonathan, and John Whalen
    1995   *Fifty Greatest Conspiracies of All Time.* New York: Carol Publishing Group.

Wadawareva, Lawrence
    1992   America Is To Blame for AIDS. Letter to the Editor. *The Chronicle* (Bulawayo). July 9. P. 5.

Waldby, Catherine and Annette Houlihan, June Crawford, and Susan Kippax
    2005   Medical Vectors: Surgical HIV Transmission and the Location of Culpability. *Sexuality Research and Social Policy* 2(2):23–30.

Walker, Deward E.
    1989   Introduction. In *Witchcraft and Sorcery of the American Native Peoples.* Walker, Deward E., ed., pp. 1–10. Moscow: Idaho.

Walters, D. W.
    1980   Runyoka or Rukawo. *NADA, The Rhodesia Ministry Internal Affairs Annual* 12(2):150–53.

Warwick, I., P. Aggleton, and H. Homans
    1988   Constructing Commonsense, Young Persons' Beliefs About AIDS. *Sociology of Health and Illness* 10:213–33.

Washington, Tawana C.
    1998   *Risk, Conspiracy, AIDS/HIV, and the African American Community: The Interaction of Trust, Control, Involvement, and Uncertainty.* M.A. School of Communication. University of Houston.

Waters, Anita
    1997   Conspiracy Theories as Ethnosociologies: Explanations and Intentions in African American Political Culture. *Journal of Black Studies* 28(1):112–25.

Watts, Ronald
    1994   AIDS and Biological Warfare Connection. *The Sunday Mail* (Harare). July 31, p. 9.

Webb, Douglas
    1997   *HIV and AIDS in Africa.* London: Pluto Press.

Weiss, Robin A.
    2003   HIV and AIDS in Relation to Other Pandemics. *European Molecular Biology Organization Reports* 4 (Special Issue): 10–14.

Wekwete, K.
    1987   *Development of Urban Planning in Zimbabwe, An Overview.* RUP Occasional Papers: Volume 8. Harare: Department of Rural and Urban Planning at the University of Zimbabwe.

Wermter, Oskar
    2003   If You Smell a Witch You Are One Yourself. *The Daily News* (Harare). July 23, p. 8.

West, Harry G.
2003   "Who Rules Us Now?" Identity Tokens, Sorcery, and Other Metaphors in the 1994 Mozambican Elections. In *Transparency and Conspiracy: Ethnographies of Suspicion in the New World Order.* West, Harry G., and Todd Sanders, eds., pp. 92–124. Durham: Duke University Press.

West, Michael O.
1994   Nationalism, Race, and Gender: The Politics of Family Planning in Zimbabwe: 1957-1990. *Social History of Medicine* 7(3):447–71.

Westerlund, David
1989   Introduction: Indigenous Pluralism and Multiple Medical Systems. In *Culture, Experience, and Pluralism: Essays on African Ideas of Illness and Healing.* A. Jacobson-Widding and D. Westerlund, eds., pp. 169–218. Acta Universitatis Upsaliensis, Vol. 13. Uppsala: University of Uppsala.

Whetten-Goldstein, Kathryn and Trang Quyen Nguyen
2002   *"You are the First One I've Told": New Faces of HIV in the South.* New Brunswick: Rutgers University Press.

White, Luise
2000   *Speaking with Vampires: Rumor and History in Colonial Africa.* Studies on the History of Society and Culture: Volume 37. Berkeley: University of California Press.
2004   Poisoned Food, Poisoned Uniforms, and Anthrax: Or, How Guerillas Die in War. *Osiris* 19:220–33.

Whitehead, Neil L.
2002   *Dark Shamans: Kanaimà and the Poetics of Violent Death.* Durham: Duke University Press.

Whiteside, Alan
1993   The Impact of AIDS on Industry in Zimbabwe. In *Facing up to AIDS: The Socio-economic Impact in Southern Africa.* S. Cross and A. Whitehead, eds., pp. 217–40. Houndmills: Macmillan.

Willis, Roy
1996   Witchcraft and Sorcery. In *Encyclopedia of Social and Cultural Anthropology.* A. Barnard and J. Spencer, eds., pp. 562–64. London: Routledge.

Wilson, D., S. Msimanga, and David W. Greenspan
1988   Knowledge About AIDS and Self-Reported Sexual Behavior Among Adults in Bulawayo, Zimbabwe. *Central African Journal of Medicine* 34(5):95–97.

Wilson, Robert Anton, and Miriam Joan Hill
1998   *Everything Is Under Control: Conspiracies, Cults, and Cover-ups.* New York: HarperCollins.

Wines, Michael
2004   With Health System in Tatters, Zimbabwe Stands Defenseless. Electronic Source: http://www.nytimes.com. Last Accessed: February 5, 2004.

Wittman, A.
1933   *Die Gestalt der Hexe in der deutschen Sage.* Bruchsal: Verlag Regionalkultur.

Wolf, Angelika
    1996a   Neue Perspektiven in der Diskussion um AIDS, Die Bedeutung der Essensmetapher in Malawi. *Curare* 19(1):151–55.
    1996b   Essensmetaphern im Kontext von AIDS und Hexerei in Malawi. In *Die gesellschaftliche Konstruktion von Befindlichkeit.* A. Wolf and M. Stürzer, eds., pp. 205–221. Berlin: Verlag für Wissenschaft und Bildung.
Woudenberg, van Judith
    1998   *Women Coping with HIV/AIDS: We Take It as It Is.* Bulletins of the Royal Tropical Institute: Volume 344. Amsterdam: Royal Tropical Institute.
Wright, Pearce
    1987   Smallpox Vaccine Triggered AIDS Virus. *The Times* (London). May 11, p. 1.
Yamba, Bawa C.
    1997   Cosmologies in Turmoil: Witchfinding and AIDS in Chiawa, Zambia. *Africa* 67(2):200–223.
Young, T. J.
    1990   Cult Violence and the Identity Movement. *Cultic Studies Journal* 7:150–59.
Zhakata, Andrew
    1992   Traditional and Bizarre Way of Discouraging Adultery. *The Chronicle* (Bulawayo). May 9. P. 4.
Zimbabwe Human Rights NGO Forum
    2001a   *Organized Violence and Torture in Zimbabwe in 2000.* Harare: Zimbabwe Human Rights NGO Forum.
    2001b   *Politically Motivated Violence in Zimbabwe 2000–2001: A Report on the Campaign of Political Repression Conducted by the Zimbabwean Government under the Guise of Carrying out Land Reform.* Harare: Zimbabwe Human Rights NGO Forum.
    2002   *Are They Accountable? Examining Alleged Violators and Their Violations Pre and Post the Presidential Election March 2002.* Harare: Zimbabwe Human Rights NGO Forum.
    2003   *Zimbabwe, the Abuja Agreement and Commonwealth Principles: Compliance or Disregard?* Harare: Zimbabwe Human Rights NGO Forum.
Zonis, Marvin, and Craig M. Joseph
    1994   Conspiracy Thinking in the Middle East. *Political Psychology* 15(3):443–59.
Zukier, Henri
    1987   The Conspirational Imperative: Medieval Jewry in Western Europe. In *Changing Conceptions of Conspiracy.* C. F. Graumann and S. Moscovici, eds., pp. 87–103. Springer Series in Social Psychology. New York: Springer-Verlag.

Index

Page numbers in *italics* refer to illustrations.

T
taboos, 21, 129–132
See also inhlonipho; social norms
taxes: to combat AIDS, 39–40
theft: by familiars, 75
Tonga (ethnic group), 36, 103n3
townships, 37, 47n3
Traditional Medical Practitioner's Act
(1981), 33n9
traditional medicine. *See under* medicine
travel: and AIDS, 64
See also migrant laborers
treatment of AIDS, 13
See also aid agencies
trust: of aid agencies, 183–184, 185
in fieldwork, 21–22, 27–28, 176
Tshuma, Zephania (artist), 32n1
Tuskegee Project, 115, 118, 137

U
ulunyoka (Ndebele; magical substance),
63, 87, *100,* 173
and AIDS, 101–102
as deterrent, 92, 94
ingredients for, 99
method of use, 53, 90
symptoms of, 99, 100, *100,* 104n12
and Tonga (ethnic group), 103n3
treatment for, 100–101
used to influence behavior, 88, 89–90,
91–92
See also infidelity; *isidliso* (sorcery
poison); poisons and poisoning;
promiscuity
umkhoba (Ndebele; sorcerer's familiar), 74
umthakathi (Ndebele; sorcerer or witch),
52
umuthi ("medicine"), 25, 144, 154
ambiguity of, 25, 32n7, 74
compared to AIDS, 164
and condoms, 151
undertakers: as conspirators, 136, 138,
139
undofa (familiar; pl. *ondofa*), 53, 73–74,
75, 173
and AIDS, 81, 82, 83–84
appearance of, 74–75, 85n3
behavior of, 73–74, 75, 76, 77–78,
85n3
and blood, 74, 77–78, 81–82

effect on spouse, 63, 79
means of repelling, 78–79
and migrant laborers, 75–76, 79–80
and sex, 79, 80–81, 83
and successful men, 57, 62
symptoms of abuse by, 81–82
risks of using, 76–77
used to accumulate wealth, 73, 75
used to punish enemies, 73
visibility of, 73–74
See also sorcery
unemployment, 45, 60
United Kingdom, 36, 144, 146
United States government, 118–119, 122
See also conspiracy theories; race and
racism

V
vaccinations, 149–150
values, 186–187
in bestiality narratives, 162, 167
loss of, 131–132, 147–148
See also infidelity; metaphors;
promiscuity; social norms
vampires: *ondofa* as, 77–78, 81–82
Venda (ethnic group), 36
venereal disease, 161, 167; *See also* AIDS
veterans. *See* soldiers and veterans
visual anthropology, 19

W
wards: politics in, 37–38
warfare: and majority rule, 142, 145–146
See also colonialism
water: poisoning of, 153
to repel *ondofa,* 78–79
weakness: and poisoning, 100
wealth: and familiars, 73, 75
and sorcery, 57, 61–62, 70n18, 70n20
See also greed and selfishness; *undofa*
Westerners: as cause of AIDS, 114, 141, 145
greed of, 143–144
See also Americans; race and racism
wheelbarrows: as transport, 30, 33n14
whites. *See* Americans; blame; Europeans;
race and racism; Westerners
witchcraft, 15n2, 52, 69n4, 85n8
See also sorcery
Witchcraft Suppression Act of 1899, 26,
33n9

About the Author

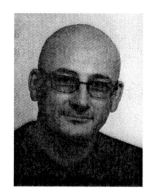

Alexander Rödlach was born in Innsbruck, Austria. Having completed his studies of philosophy and theology with distinction, he received in 1990 the *Baccalaureatus Theologiae* (*magna cum laude*) from the Pontificia Università Urbaniana in Rome, Italy, and the *Magister der Theologie* from the Theologische Hochschule St. Gabriel, Mödling, Austria. He was then ordained a priest in the Society of the Divine Word and worked from 1991 to 1998 as a missionary in Plumtree and Bulawayo, Zimbabwe. From 1998 to 2005 he did graduate studies in anthropology, first at the Catholic University of America in Washington, DC, and then at the University of Florida, Gainesville, concluding with a doctorate. He currently works at the Anthropos Institute, St. Augustine, in the editorial department of *Anthropos*.

Rödlach is the author of several articles and book chapters including "Religious Beliefs at the Service of Nationalist Politics in Joshua Nkomo's Writings" (*Verbum* [42]1: 49–79); "Apocalypse Now! Interpretations of HIV/AIDS in an Urban Township in Bulawayo, Zimbabwe" (In Lazar, Imre and Agita Luse, eds.); and *Cosmologies of Suffering* (Newcastle-upon-Tyne: Cambridge Scholars Press [in press]).